Breast Imaging

Editor

PHOEBE E. FREER

RADIOLOGIC CLINICS
OF NORTH AMERICA

www.radiologic.theclinics.com

Consulting Editor
FRANK H. MILLER

January 2021 • Volume 59 • Number 1

ELSEVIER

1600 John F. Kennedy Boulevard • Suite 1800 • Philadelphia, Pennsylvania, 19103-2899

http://www.theclinics.com

RADIOLOGIC CLINICS OF NORTH AMERICA Volume 59, Number 1
January 2021 ISSN 0033-8389, ISBN 13: 978-0-323-76477-3

Editor: John Vassallo (j.vassallo@elsevier.com)
Developmental Editor: Donald Mumford

Radiologic Clinics of North America (ISSN 0033-8389) is published bimonthly by Elsevier Inc., 360 Park Avenue South, New York, NY 10010-1710. Months of issue are January, March, May, July, September, and November. Periodicals postage paid at New York, NY and additional mailing offices. Subscription prices are USD 518 per year for US individuals, USD 1309 per year for US institutions, USD 100 per year for US students and residents, USD 611 per year for Canadian individuals, USD 1368 per year for Canadian institutions, USD 703 per year for international individuals, USD 1368 per year for international institutions, USD 100 per year for Canadian students/residents, and USD 315 per year for international students/residents. To receive student and resident rate, orders must be accompanied by name of affiliated institution, date of term and the signature of program/residency coordinatior on institution letterhead. Orders will be billed at individual rate until proof of status is received. Foreign air speed delivery is included in all *Clinics* subscription prices. All prices are subject to change without notice. **POSTMASTER:** Send address changes to *Radiologic Clinics of North America*, Elsevier Health Sciences Division, Subscription Customer Service, 3251 Riverport Lane, Maryland Heights, MO63043. **Customer Service: Telephone: 1-800-654-2452** (U.S. and Canada); **1-314-447-8871** (outside U.S. and Canada). **Fax: 1-314-447-8029. E-mail: journalscustomerservice-usa@elsevier.com (for print support); journalsonlinesupport-usa@elsevier.com (for online support)**.

Reprints. For copies of 100 or more of articles in this publication, please contact the Commercial Reprints Department, Elsevier Inc., 360 Park Avenue South, New York, New York 10010-1710. Tel.: +1-212-633-3874; Fax: +1-212-633-3820; E-mail: reprints@elsevier.com.

Radiologic Clinics of North America also published in Greek Paschalidis Medical Publications, Athens, Greece.

Radiologic Clinics of North America is covered in *MEDLINE/PubMed (Index Medicus), EMBASE/Excerpta Medica, Current Contents/Life Sciences, Current Contents/Clinical Medicine, RSNA Index to Imaging Literature, BIOSIS, Science Citation Index,* and *ISI/BIOMED.*

Contributors

CONSULTING EDITOR

FRANK H. MILLER, MD, FACR
Lee F. Rogers MD Professor of Medical
Education, Chief, Body Imaging Section and
Fellowship Program, Medical Director, MRI,
Department of Radiology, Northwestern
Memorial Hospital, Northwestern University,
Feinberg School of Medicine, Chicago, Illinois,
USA

EDITOR

PHOEBE E. FREER, MD, FSBI
Section Chief, Breast Imaging, Associate
Professor of Radiology, Department of
Radiology and Imaging Sciences, University of
Utah Health/Huntsman Cancer Institute, Salt
Lake City, Utah, USA

AUTHORS

DANA ATAYA, MD
Assistant Member, Department of Diagnostic
Imaging and Interventional Radiology,
Assistant Professor, Department of Oncologic
Sciences, University of South Florida, H. Lee
Moffitt Cancer Center and Research Institute,
Tampa, Florida, USA

MANISHA BAHL, MD, MPH
Assistant Professor of Radiology, Harvard
Medical School, Radiologist, Massachusetts
General Hospital, Boston, Massachusetts,
USA

DEBBIE L. BENNETT, MD
Department of Radiology, Washington
University School of Medicine, St Louis,
Missouri, USA

ALMIR G.V. BITENCOURT, MD, PhD
Breast Imaging Service, Department of
Radiology, Memorial Sloan Kettering Cancer
Center, New York, New York, USA;

Department of Imaging, A.C. Camargo Cancer
Center, São Paulo, São Paulo, Brazil

MATTHEW F. COVINGTON, MD
Assistant Professor of Breast Imaging and
Nuclear Medicine, Department of Radiology
and Imaging Sciences, University of Utah,
Center for Quantitative Cancer Imaging,
Huntsman Cancer Institute, Salt Lake City,
Utah, USA

PHOEBE E. FREER, MD, FSBI
Section Chief, Breast Imaging, Associate
Professor of Radiology, Department of
Radiology and Imaging Sciences, University of
Utah Health/Huntsman Cancer Institute, Salt
Lake City, Utah, USA

KIMBERLY FUNARO, MD
Assistant Member, Department of Diagnostic
Imaging and Interventional Radiology,
Assistant Professor, Department of Oncologic
Sciences, University of South Florida, H. Lee

Moffitt Cancer Center and Research Institute, Tampa, Florida, USA

YIMING GAO, MD
Department of Radiology, NYU School of Medicine, New York, New York, USA

LAURA HEACOCK, MS, MD
Clinical Assistant Professor, Department of Radiology, NYU Grossman School of Medicine, New York, New York, USA

SAMANTHA L. HELLER, PhD, MD
Department of Radiology, NYU School of Medicine, New York, New York, USA

MARK A. HELVIE, MD
Professor, Department of Radiology, Breast Imaging Division, University of Michigan, Ann Arbor, Michigan, USA

DIANA L. LAM, MD
Assistant Professor, Department of Radiology, University of Washington School of Medicine, Seattle, Washington, USA

JANIE M. LEE, MD, MSc
Professor, Department of Radiology, University of Washington School of Medicine, Seattle, Washington, USA

ALANA A. LEWIN, MD
Clinical Assistant Professor, Department of Radiology, NYU Grossman School of Medicine, New York, New York, USA

JONATHAN L. MATES, MD
Medical Director of Product, Viz.ai, San Francisco, California, USA

MATTHEW B. MORGAN, MD, MS
Associate Professor of Radiology, Department of Radiology and Imaging Sciences, University of Utah, Salt Lake City, Utah, USA

ELIZABETH A. MORRIS, MD
Chief, Breast Imaging Service, Department of Radiology, Memorial Sloan Kettering Cancer Center, New York, New York, USA

LINDA MOY, MD
Professor, Department of Radiology, NYU Grossman School of Medicine, Center for

Biomedical Imaging, Center for Advanced Imaging Innovation and Research, New York, New York, USA

COLLEEN H. NEAL, MD
Clinical Associate Professor, Department of Radiology, Breast Imaging Division, University of Michigan, Ann Arbor, Michigan, USA

BETHANY NIELL, MD, PhD
Associate Member, Department of Diagnostic Imaging and Interventional Radiology, Associate Professor, Breast Imaging Section Chief, Department of Oncologic Sciences, University of South Florida, H. Lee Moffitt Cancer Center and Research Institute, Tampa, Florida, USA

AMY K. PATEL, MD
Medical Director, Liberty Hospital Women's Imaging, Alliance Radiology, Department of Radiology, University of Missouri-Kansas City School of Medicine, Liberty, Missouri, USA

BEATRIU REIG, MD, MPH
Clinical Assistant Professor, Department of Radiology, NYU Grossman School of Medicine, New York, New York, USA

CAROLINA ROSSI SACCARELLI, MD
Breast Imaging Service, Department of Radiology, Memorial Sloan Kettering Cancer Center, New York, New York, USA; Department of Radiology, Hospital Sírio-Libanês, São Paulo, São Paulo, Brazil

ROBERTA M. STRIGEL, MD, MS
Associate Professor of Radiology and Medical Physics, Section Chief, Breast Imaging and Intervention, University of Wisconsin, Madison, Wisconsin, USA

HILDEGARD K. TOTH, MD
Professor, Department of Radiology, NYU Grossman School of Medicine, New York, New York, USA

LILIAN WANG, MD
Assistant Professor of Radiology, Northwestern Medicine, Prentice Women's Hospital, Chicago, Illinois, USA

Contents

The Covid-19 pandemic of 2020 caused great disruption to breast imaging and breast cancer care. Screening mammography was deferred nationwide (and internationally) for a period of weeks to months. Patients and some breast centers delayed diagnostic imaging and biopsies leading to a decrease in the incidence of cancer detected. Additionally, there were significant changes to breast cancer care algorithms. Practices were greatly affected financially as well as in terms of workflow logistics and educational methods. The many reaching effects of the pandemic on breast imaging are reviewed.

In an increasingly competitive and passionate health care environment, radiology advocacy is imperative, now more than ever. Arguably, it is particularly more crucial in the world of breast cancer, as we as a breast cancer community are tirelessly assembling to advocate for our patients on a variety of levels, whether it is including but not limited to, breast cancer screening, diagnosis, and treatment, access-to-care, education, or research funding. As breast radiologists, it is no longer simply enough to clock in our normal work hours; we must ALL make a concerted effort to vociferously advocate for our patients and profession.

Since its widespread introduction 30 years ago, screening mammography has contributed to substantial reduction in breast cancer-associated mortality, ranging from 15% to 50% in observational trials. It is currently the best examination available for the early diagnosis of breast cancer, when survival and treatment options are most favorable. However, like all medical tests and procedures, screening mammography has associated risks, including overdiagnosis and overtreatment, false-positive examinations, false-positive biopsies, and radiation exposure. Women should be aware of the benefits and risks of screening mammography in order to make the most appropriate care decisions for themselves.

High-risk breast lesions (HRLs) are a group of heterogeneous lesions that can be associated with a synchronous or adjacent breast cancer and that confer an elevated lifetime risk of breast cancer. Management of HRLs after core needle biopsy may include close imaging and clinical follow-up or excisional biopsy to evaluate for cancer. This article reviews histologic features and clinical presentation of each of the HRLs, current evidence with regard to management, and guidelines from the American Society of Breast Surgeons and National Comprehensive Cancer Network. In addition, imaging surveillance and risk-reduction strategies for women with HRLs are discussed.

Screening mammography aims to identify small, node-negative breast cancers when they are still curable while maintaining an acceptable range of false-positive recalls and biopsies. The mammography audit is a powerful tool to help radiologists understand their performance with respect to that goal. This article defines audit terms and describes how to use collected and derived data to perform a mammography audit. Accepted benchmarks are discussed as well as their applicability to radiologists and breast imaging practices in the United States. Special considerations regarding volumes and radiologist characteristics are explored, because these factors may affect audit results.

Breast magnetic resonance (MR) imaging is the most sensitive imaging modality for breast cancer detection and guidelines recommend its use, in addition to screening mammography, for high-risk women. The most recent American College of Radiology (ACR) Breast Imaging Reporting and Data System (BI-RADS) manual coordinated cross-modality BI-RADS terminology and established an outcome monitoring section that helps guide a medical imaging outcomes audit. This article provides a framework for performing a breast MR imaging audit in clinical practice, incorporating ACR BI-RADS guidance and more recently published data, clarifies common pitfalls, and discusses audit challenges related to evolving clinical practice.

The sensitivity of mammography is more limited in patients with dense breasts and some patients at higher risk for breast cancer. Patients with intermediate or high risk for breast cancer may begin screening earlier and benefit from supplemental screening techniques beyond standard 2-dimensional mammography. A patient's individual risk factors for developing breast cancer, their breast density, and the evidence supporting specific modalities for a given clinical scenario help to determine the need for supplemental screening and the modality chosen. Additional factors include the availability of supplemental screening techniques at an individual institution, cost, insurance coverage, and state-specific breast density legislation.

Magnetic Resonance (MR) imaging is the most sensitive modality for breast cancer detection but is currently limited to screening women at high risk due to limited specificity and test accessibility. However, specificity of MR imaging improves with successive rounds of screening, and abbreviated approaches have the potential to increase access and decrease cost. There is growing evidence to support supplemental MR imaging in moderate-risk women, and current guidelines continue to evolve. Functional imaging has the potential to maximize survival benefit of screening. Leveraging MR imaging as a possible primary screening tool is therefore also being investigated in average-risk women.

Laura Heacock, Alana A. Lewin, Hildegard K. Toth, Linda Moy, and Beatriu Reig

Breast MR imaging is the most sensitive imaging method for the detection of breast cancer and detects more aggressive malignancies than mammography and ultrasound examination. Despite these advantages, breast MR imaging has low use rates for breast cancer screening. Abbreviated breast MR imaging, in which a limited number of breast imaging sequences are obtained, has been proposed as a way to solve cost and patient tolerance issues while preserving the high cancer detection rate of breast MR imaging. This review discusses abbreviated breast MR imaging, including protocols, multicenter clinical trial results, clinical workflow implementation challenges, and future directions.

Matthew F. Covington

Contrast-enhanced mammography (CEM) is an emerging breast imaging technology that provides recombined contrast-enhanced images of the breast in addition to low-energy images analogous to a 2-dimensional full-field digital mammogram. Because most breast imaging centers do not use CEM at this time, a detailed overview of CEM implementation and performance is presented. Thereafter, the potential use of CEM for supplemental screening is discussed in detail, given the importance of this topic for the future of the CEM community. Diagnostic performance, safety, and cost considerations of CEM for dense breast tissue supplemental screening are discussed.

Carolina Rossi Saccarelli, Almir G.V. Bitencourt, and Elizabeth A. Morris

Breast cancer screening is a recognized tool for early detection of the disease in asymptomatic women, improving treatment efficacy and reducing the mortality rate. There is raised awareness that a "one-size-fits-all" approach cannot be applied for breast cancer screening. Currently, despite specific guidelines for a minority of women who are at very high risk of breast cancer, all other women are still treated alike. This article reviews the current recommendations for breast cancer risk assessment and breast cancer screening in average-risk and higher-than-average-risk women. Also discussed are new developments and future perspectives for personalized breast cancer screening.

Matthew B. Morgan and Jonathan L. Mates

Artificial intelligence (AI) technology shows promise in breast imaging to improve both interpretive and noninterpretive tasks. AI-based screening triage may help identify normal examinations and AI-based computer-aided detection (AI-CAD) may increase cancer detection and reduce false positives. Risk assessment, quality assurance, and other workflow tasks may also be streamlined. AI adoption will depend on robust evidence of improved quality, increased efficiency, and cost-effectiveness. Reliance on AI will likely proceed through stages and will involve careful attention to its limitations to prevent overconfidence in its application.

PROGRAM OBJECTIVE

The objective of the *Radiologic Clinics of North America* is to keep practicing radiologists and radiology residents up to date with current clinical practice in radiology by providing timely articles reviewing the state of the art in patient care.

TARGET AUDIENCE

Practicing radiologists, radiology residents, and other healthcare professionals who provide patient care utilizing radiologic findings.

LEARNING OBJECTIVES

Upon completion of this activity, participants will be able to:
1. Describe implications and effects of the COVID-19 pandemic on breast imaging.
2. Discuss the risks of screening and overdiagnosis of breast cancer.
3. Recognize the importance of radiologist advocacy in regard to breast cancer screening, supplemental screening, and the timing of screening.

ACCREDITATION

The Elsevier Office of Continuing Medical Education (EOCME) is accredited by the Accreditation Council for Continuing Medical Education (ACCME) to provide continuing medical education for physicians.

The EOCME designates this journal-based CME activity for a maximum of 11 *AMA PRA Category 1 Credit*(s)™. Physicians should claim only the credit commensurate with the extent of their participation in the activity.

All other healthcare professionals requesting continuing education credit for this enduring material will be issued a certificate of participation.

DISCLOSURE OF CONFLICTS OF INTEREST

The EOCME assesses conflict of interest with its instructors, faculty, planners, and other individuals who are in a position to control the content of CME activities. All relevant conflicts of interest that are identified are thoroughly vetted by EOCME for fair balance, scientific objectivity, and patient care recommendations. EOCME is committed to providing its learners with CME activities that promote improvements or quality in healthcare and not a specific proprietary business or a commercial interest.

The planning committee, staff, authors and editors listed below have identified no financial relationships or relationships to products or devices they or their spouse/life partner have with commercial interest related to the content of this CME activity:

Dana Ataya, MD; Manisha Bahl, MD, MPH; Debbie L. Bennett, MD; Almir G.V. Bitencourt, MD, PhD; Regina Chavous-Gibson, MSN, RN; Phoebe E. Freer, MD, FSBI; Kimberly Funaro, MD; Yiming Gao, MD; Laura Heacock, MS, MD; Samantha L. Heller, PhD, MD; Pradeep Kuttysankaran; Diana L. Lam, MD; Alana A. Lewin, MD; Linda Moy, MD; Colleen H. Neal, MD; Bethany Niell, MD, PhD; Amy K. Patel, MD; Beatriu Reig, MD, MPH; Carolina Rossi Saccarelli, MD; Hildegard K. Toth, MD; John Vassallo; Lilian Wang, MD

The planning committee, staff, authors and editors listed below have identified financial relationships or relationships to products or devices they or their spouse/life partner have with commercial interest related to the content of this CME activity:

Matthew F. Covington, MD: consultant/advisor for Hologic, Inc.

Mark A. Helvie, MD: research support from General Electric Company

Janie M. Lee, MD, MSc: research support from General Electric Company

Jonathan L. Mates, MD: employment with Viz.ai, Inc.

Matthew B. Morgan, MD, MS: consultant/advisor at Elsevier

Elizabeth A. Morris, MD: research support from Grail, Inc.

Roberta M. Strigel, MD, MS: research support from General Electric Company

UNAPPROVED/OFF-LABEL USE DISCLOSURE

The EOCME requires CME faculty to disclose to the participants:
1. When products or procedures being discussed are off-label, unlabelled, experimental, and/or investigational (not US Food and Drug Administration [FDA] approved); and
2. Any limitations on the information presented, such as data that are preliminary or that represent ongoing research, interim analyses, and/or unsupported opinions. Faculty may discuss information about pharmaceutical agents that is outside of FDA-approved labelling. This information is intended solely for CME and is not intended to promote off-label use of these medications. If you have any questions, contact the medical affairs department of the manufacturer for the most recent prescribing information.

TO ENROLL

To enroll in the *Radiologic Clinics of North America* Continuing Medical Education program, call customer service at 1-800-654-2452 or sign up online at http://www.theclinics.com/home/cme. The CME program is available to subscribers for an additional annual fee of USD 356.00.

METHOD OF PARTICIPATION

In order to claim credit, participants must complete the following:

1. Complete enrolment as indicated above.
2. Read the activity.
3. Complete the CME Test and Evaluation. Participants must achieve a score of 70% on the test. All CME Tests and Evaluations must be completed online.

CME INQUIRIES/SPECIAL NEEDS

For all CME inquiries or special needs, please contact elsevierCME@elsevier.com.

RADIOLOGIC CLINICS OF NORTH AMERICA

RELATED SERIES

Advances in Clinical Radiology
www.advancesinclinicalradiology.com
MRI Clinics
www.mri.theclinics.com
Neuroimaging Clinics
www.neuroimaging.theclinics.com
PET Clinics
www.pet.theclinics.com

THE CLINICS ARE AVAILABLE ONLINE!
Access your subscription at:
www.theclinics.com

RADIOLOGIC CLINICS OF NORTH AMERICA

Preface
An Emerging Era for Breast Imaging

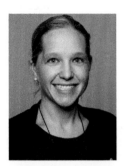

Phoebe E. Freer, MD, FSBI

Editor

This issue was prepared amid a once-in-a-lifetime pandemic from COVID-19. At the time of writing this preface, there were nearly 30 million cases with almost 1 million deaths worldwide and over 6.5 million cases in the United States.[1] The pandemic affected public health, including breast imaging algorithms, greatly. Mammographic screening came to a near complete halt for a short time period in March / April 2020 with a slow reemergence over the next few months. It also disrupted diagnostic breast imaging and cancer care algorithms. The implications and effects of the pandemic on breast imaging, care algorithms, outcomes, and radiologists are reviewed in 1 article in this issue, as some effects will likely be practice changing in the long term. The articles in this issue were written amid the pandemic turmoil, with significant disruptions in many of the authors' daily lives secondary to the pandemic. I extend a heartfelt thank you to contributors juggling academic and educational pursuits during such a time.

Nevertheless, breast imaging remains of paramount importance in cancer care. As debates regarding breast cancer screening, supplemental screening, and the timing of screening continue to evolve, this issue highlights the importance of radiologist advocacy with a call to action. Another article reviews the risks of screening, most importantly with a thorough review of the evidence regarding overdiagnosis and how best to assess measurements of overdiagnosis. Screening may find high-risk lesions and subsequently change a patient's underlying risk for breast cancer in terms of risk stratifying for supplemental screening, and thus a review of the management of high-risk breast lesions is included. When evaluating screening and supplemental screening, a good understanding of the audit is required, and as such, articles discussing the nuances of the mammography audit and the MR imaging audit are included. Several evidence-based up-to-date articles on supplemental screening in high-risk women or in dense breasts are included that discuss emerging and recent literature. These include an overall review of supplemental screening as well as reviews of MR imaging and abbreviated MR imaging for screening and contrast-enhanced mammography. Given

Radiol Clin N Am 59 (2021) xiii–xiv
https://doi.org/10.1016/j.rcl.2020.09.007
0033-8389/21/© 2020 Published by Elsevier Inc.

the evolving evidence on supplemental screening techniques and a better understanding of the risks of screening, an article addresses the question of whether screening remains a one-size-fits-all approach or should be more personalized. Finally, given the large cultural and scientific focus on artificial intelligence and developing algorithms for improved care, an article on artificial intelligence in breast imaging is included.

I hope that both experts and trainees may find pearls to learn from in these pages and will find this issue a valuable and relevant update to the literature on breast imaging. I am grateful so many extraordinary leaders and emerging leaders in the field contributed, especially during these times.

Phoebe E. Freer, MD, FSBI
University of Utah Radiology
University of Utah Hospital
50 2030 E
Salt Lake City, UT 84132, USA

E-mail address:
phoebe.freer@hsc.utah.edu

REFERENCE

1. Coronavirus Resource Center. Johns Hopkins University School of Medicine. Available at: https://coronavirus.jhu.edu. Accessed September 16, 2020.

The Impact of the COVID-19 Pandemic on Breast Imaging

Phoebe E. Freer, MD, FSBI

KEYWORDS

- COVID-19 • Pandemic • Breast cancer • Breast imaging • Delayed care • Radiology finances

KEY POINTS

- The COVID-19 pandemic starting in the United States in 2020 has had practice-changing effects on cancer care, clinical workflow, education, research, and radiology finances.
- Significant volume reductions and delays occurred to breast imaging, with screening mammography being the hardest hit.
- Long-term outcomes from changes in breast cancer management algorithm during the pandemic are yet to be determined.
- Increased telehealth and telecommuting will likely continue after the pandemic is over in some fashion.
- Radiology practices and hospitals sustained large financial ramifications from the effects of the pandemic.

INTRODUCTION

Starting in Wuhan, China, followed quickly in the United States in January 2020, an outbreak of a novel coronavirus, or COVID-19, escalated to a global pandemic by March. Significant disruptions occurred to breast imaging, including deferred screening mammography, triaging diagnostic breast imaging, and changes in breast cancer care algorithms. This article summarizes the effect of the global pandemic—and efforts to curtail its spread—on both breast cancer care and on breast imaging practices including effects on patients, clinical workflow, education, and research.

INITIAL RESPONSE: ROUTINE HEALTH CARE DEFERRED

The approach to the handling of COVID-19 has been fluid, as understanding of the pathophysiology, clinical spectrum and severity of illness, and possible preventions and treatment of the virus have evolved.[1,2]

Early Response: Concerns for Mammography in COVID-19

Shortly after the first outbreaks in the United States on the Diamond Princess Cruise Ship, in Seattle and New York, on the heels of large outbreaks in China and Italy, the main prevention strategy of "social distancing" was adopted by the World Health Organization.[3] By April 2020, 33 states had state mandated "stay-at-home-orders." The Centers for Disease control (CDC) issued recommendations to reschedule nonurgent patient care and delay screenings in an effort to minimize risks to patients and health care workers (HCWs).[4] Although social distancing measures varied regionally, most of the school systems, churches, and businesses were closed in March or April 2020, often moving to virtual encounters. Leaders in breast imaging and radiology departments discussed the best ways to protect patients, protect HCWs, and conserve personal protective equipment (PPE) and ventilators to be

Breast Imaging, Department of Radiology and Imaging Sciences, University of Utah Health / Huntsman Cancer Institute, 30 North 1900 East #1A071, Salt Lake City, UT 84132, USA
E-mail address: Phoebe.Freer@hsc.utah.edu

Radiol Clin N Am 59 (2021) 1–11
https://doi.org/10.1016/j.rcl.2020.09.008
0033-8389/21/© 2020 Elsevier Inc. All rights reserved.

used for patients with COVID-19.[5] Many sites began rescheduling screening mammography patients, some diagnostic or biopsy cases, or even delaying breast surgeries in an ad hoc fashion. Varied interpretations of the CDC, WHO, and the varied state policies led to nonuniform disruptions in patient care, in some cases varying within the same large cities.[6]

On March 24th, news reports of potential danger to mammography technologists from work exposures were released, with a death of a mammography technologist in Georgia from COVID-19, a possible work exposure.[7] HCWs were confirmed to be high risk for COVID-19 infections (up to 10%) from initial data in early outbreaks in China, Italy, and Spain.[8] The *National Comprehensive Cancer Network* (NCCN) issued guidelines for health care worker safety early in the pandemic, based on WHO recommendations.[9] In a study rating different professions' risk of contracting COVID-19 from work, radiology technologists were one of the highest (a score or 84 out of 100), and then sonographers (80 out of 100).[10] Mammography technologists likely have an even higher risk, as they are unable to maintain social distancing (2 m or 6 feet) during positioning.

Quickly, breast radiologists and technologists had palpable concerns regarding the need to protect HCWs and patients during screening, and firm statements were released by national organizations with the American Society of Breast Surgeons (ASBrS) and American College of Radiology (ACR) Joint Statement on Breast Screening Exams During the COVID-19 Pandemic and the Society of Breast Imaging Statement on Breast Imaging during the COVID-19 Pandemic, all released later in March, 2020, and recommending to "postpone all breast screening exams (to include screening mammography, ultrasound, and MRI) effective immediately" as well as to discontinue routine and nonurgent breast health appointments.[11,12]

Moreover, shortages of PPE existed, and so technologist and radiologists could not uniformly be masked, with only 35.3% (60 of 170) of radiology practices stating they had an adequate supply and 29.4% reporting that PPE supplies were low and needed to rationed.[13]

A More Standardized Approach to Deferred Care

By March, the Canadian Society of Breast Imaging and Canadian Association of Radiologists Joint Position Statement on COVID-19 recommended that all screening mammography and MR imaging be deferred for at least 6 to 8 weeks and suggested triaging the diagnostic cases, deferring ones that were not highly suspicious for cancer.[14] The Society of Breast Imaging followed suit with a statement that was broader and less prescriptive but also recommended delaying screening by "several weeks or a few months."[15] Other international societies published similar statements.[16,17]

Multidisciplinary care algorithms changed the management of breast cancer during the pandemic in response to need to balance the urgency of care against the risks to patients and HCWs secondary to potential COVID-19 exposures. Surgeries were postponed both to limit COVID-19 transmission as well as to preserve resources such as ventilators, PPE, and hospital beds. The American College of Surgeons (ACS) and the Society of Surgical Oncology released triage guidelines recommending an interim cancellation of most routine surgeries, while still performing breast surgeries for those in more urgent cases.[18,19] Some centers, such as Magee-Breast Cancer Program and Johns Hopkins published multidisciplinary algorithms of how best to triage patients with breast cancer, broken down by subtypes.[20,21] Other published tools suggested risk-stratifying patients for breast surgery with the purpose of causing few deleterious effects in patients recommended for postponement.[22]

In early April, a multidisciplinary group of breast cancer experts in the United States formed the COVID-19 Pandemic Breast Cancer Consortium and released its recommendations for prioritization, treatment, and triage of patients with breast cancer during the COVID-19 pandemic. The panel represents a joint collaboration from the ASBrS, the National Accreditation Program for Breast Centers (NAPBC), the NCCN, the Commission on Cancer, and ACR.[23] The main goals of the Consortium recommendations were to "preserve hospital resources for virus-inflicted patients by deferring BC treatments without significantly compromising long-term outcomes for individual BC patients". Patients were placed into categories based on severity of symptoms or illnesses with algorithms for chemotherapy and surgery outlined based on disease process.

REOPENING OF ROUTINE CARE

By July 2020, as the pandemic proved lasting and PPE supplies improved nationwide, consensus guidelines shifted to avoid delays in care and focused instead on how to better protect patients and workers.[24] Leaders in breast cancer made evidence-based pleas to cease labeling patients with cancer as a high-risk population in order to avoid delays in their diagnosis and treatment.[25]

Numerous consensus statements and guidelines regarding how to best balance the risks of COVID-19 transmission to patients and HCWs against the risks of delaying care have been published.[26] The European Society for Medical Oncology Guidelines include increasing telehealth appointments (noting in person visits are needed for new patients with cancer or urgent infections/postoperative complications) and specific guidance for management and advised that the risk/benefit balance for most patients favored continued administration of systemic therapies and chemotherapies, with additional precautions when possible (eg, choosing less immunosuppressive therapies, regimens requiring fewer appointments).[25] Numerous other guidance documents have emerged fluidly including from American Society of Clinical Oncology (ASCO) and an online resource from ASCO, and others globally.[17,27–32]

Although the recommendations for the management of breast cancer change the order and timing of breast cancer treatments, the goals have remained to change these algorithms in ways that do not affect long-term outcomes or chances for a cure. For example, surgery should remain the primary option for small triple-negative breast cancers that did not require chemotherapy based on pre-COVID-19 algorithms.[33] In addition, patients with progressive disease on medical therapy should have surgery. Further patients who are competing their neoadjuvant regimens or patients who did not respond to neoadjuvant therapy should receive surgery.[33]

Prophylactic measures were implemented with guidance from the CDC, for protecting patients and HCWs, including social distancing where possible, masking both patients and HCWs, decreasing the number of scheduled patients, increasing space in waiting areas, and implementing disinfection protocols. Nearly all imaging centers implemented preappointment screening for symptoms of COVID-19, most requiring temperature screening at some point during the pandemic and a few even required COVID-19 negative testing before a breast interventional procedure (although many centers required COVID-19 negative testing before breast surgeries).[34]

CHANGES IN FOOD AND DRUG ADMINISTRATION INSPECTIONS DURING COVID-19

Initially, the FDA halted inspections of mammography facilities required by the Mammographic Quality Standards Act in mid-March, 2020. In addition, the ACR granted automatic extensions and halted in-person inspections for sites where accreditation was expiring.[35] As the reopening phase began, the FDA announced that it would restart inspections at facilities in locations that were not as affected by the pandemic on July 20th, although it did not actually start them then. It recommended that state inspections could start based on individual state guidance at the end of June 2020, guided by an advisory system to take into account the extent of the outbreak in that location combined with how critical the inspection would be.[36]

BREAST CANCER AS A COMORBIDITY FOR COVID-19 SEVERE OUTCOMES/FATALITIES

Initially, concern existed that patients with breast cancer, especially advanced or metastatic breast cancer, may be more susceptible to severe outcomes with COVID-19. Many of the most common chemotherapy regimens used to treat breast cancer are known to cause immunosuppression. Further, patients undergoing cancer care have more visits and therefore more exposures to HCWs and patients, potentially making them more at risk of being infected with COVID-19.[37,38] Initial studies from Wuhan, China showed worse outcomes from COVID-19 in patients with cancer and suggested caution with cancer care during the pandemic.[38–40] In one study of 1524 patients from the Wuhan outbreak, patients with cancer had more than double the risk of contracting COVID-19 than patients without (odds ratio [OR], 2.31; 95% confidence interval [CI], 1.89 to 3.02).[37] In another early study from the Wuhan experience, the relative risk of dying or being admitted to the intensive care unit with COVID-19 in patients with cancer was 5.4 (95% CI 1.8–16.2).[38] Moreover, patients with cancer had a higher relative risk of requiring intubation, across all age ranges.[38] The mortality rate of COVID-19 in patients with cancer has ranged from 11% to 28% in reported studies,[41–43] compared with the 1.4% mortality rate reported in the general population from the initial Wuhan studies.[44] However, not all patients with cancer have the same risks, as a patient with an early stage breast cancer may not have the COVID-19 risks as a patient with end-of-life stage IV breast cancer. This was confirmed by one study of 900 patients with cancer and COVID-19 that found that having active cancer that was progressing (as opposed to remission) and having a worse performance status were associated with increased risk of mortality.[43]

As the pandemic has unfolded, registries for patients with cancer and COVID-19 have been developed in an attempt to better understand the risk to patients with cancer, as initial reports on outcomes were limited to single institutional or smaller studies. An international database was established to study the risks of COVID-19 on patients with cancer from the United States, Canada, and Spain with underlying cancer (the COVID-19 and Cancer Consortium Database or CCC19).[43] And ASCO developed its own registry to be able to share data rapidly and contribute to evidence-based decision-making for patients with cancer during the pandemic.[45]

Initial reports from mid-March through mid-April of the CCC19, including more than 900 patients with cancer (21% breast cancer) and COVID-19 found that although the 30-day all-cause mortality for the entire population with cancer and COVID-19 was high, associated with both general and cancer-specific risk factors, the actual risk in patients with solid tumors (ie, breast cancer) was not significantly higher.[45] This study also confirmed recent cancer surgery did not affect the mortality rate from concurrent infections with COVID-19.[45] A large cohort study of 800 patients with cancer with COVID-19 in the United Kingdom (UK Coronavirus Cancer Monitoring Project), at a similar time frame of the pandemic, found that although the mortality rate was 28%, when adjusted for age and other comorbidities, the presence of cancer alone did not increase the mortality from COVID-19.[46] Importantly, the use of chemotherapy before COVID-19 infection did not affect mortality, neither did the use of hormonal, targeted, and, immune therapies, or radiation.[46]

Thus, although it may be possible that some patients with cancer have a propensity toward worse outcomes with COVID-19, it does not seem likely that cancer treatments such as chemotherapy, hormonal therapy, radiation, and surgery predispose patients to more serious outcomes from COVID-19. If care is taken for protective measures for the patients and HCWs as outlined in different care algorithms, breast cancer treatment should continue during the pandemic, especially in light of the unknown timeframe of the crisis.

EFFECTS OF DELAYING CARE ON PATIENTS WITH BREAST CANCER

Not only did multidisciplinary care algorithms force patients into delaying care during the pandemic but patients also self-selected to delay care. Nearly 4 out of 10 patients said the economic changes from the pandemic affected their ability to pay for medical care.[47] A survey by ACEP demonstrated almost one-third of patients (29%) delayed or avoided going to the emergency room in March/April 2020 in order to avoid COVID-19 exposures.[48] Four out of five patients were fearful of contracting the virus from a patient or HCW if they did go.[48] Greater than 81% of survey participants acknowledged practicing social distancing.[48] In an Italian study, during the height of the outbreak, there was a significant increase in patients refusing to undergo diagnostic appointments and breast biopsies at a major cancer center.[49]

In another 600 breast care patients surveyed, almost 80% stated they had routine and follow-up appointments delayed, two-thirds had reconstruction surgery delayed, and 60% had delayed diagnostic imaging.[50] Therapies that required in-person visits to the hospital (radiation, chemotherapy infusion, and surgical lumpectomies) were more likely to be delayed than those that could be obtained through telehealth appointments or a prescription pick-up.[50] Medicare and Medicaid Services and private insurers expanded telehealth benefits to patients covering increased virtual visits.[51] On average, about 30% of patients experienced delays in the mainstays of breast cancer treatment including lumpectomies, radiation therapy, and chemotherapy.[50] Breast cancer surgeries declined significantly during the early parts of the global pandemic.[52] In data from 55 breast centers in 27 states, it was noted that the average decline in breast surgery clinic appointments over the first few weeks was 21% with a nadir of 40% from baseline and a near 20% decline in new breast cancer surgery consultations in the surgery clinics.[52] Similarly, breast cancer genetics appointments declined, ranging between 25% and 30%.[52] In one study from Wuhan, China, more than half of the patients receiving radiation therapy were unable to complete their regimens during the lockdowns.[53] The pandemic increased the use of neoadjuvant and hormonal therapies before surgery, as well as increased genotypic profiling, secondary to deferrals of surgeries.[21] In another study from the Netherlands one-third of patients noted that the pandemic affected their cancer care, with most of these noting a shift to telehealth consultations.[54] Chemotherapy was also affected in about one-third of these patients.[54]

The long-term physical and psychosocial ramifications of these delays remain to be determined. One study demonstrated that more than half of the patients with cancer were concerned the delays or discontinuation of care during the pandemic affected their outcomes.[54] Oncologic patients noted anxieties regarding whether they were at increased risk of worse outcomes with COVID-19, as well as anger and worry from delays or interruptions in their care during COVID-19. Some patients even stated that the changes in their care encountered sounded "like a death sentence" or made them "feel like my care and health aren't important to you".[55] These patient perceptions, whether accurate or not, will need to be addressed as the pandemic unfolds.[55,56]

The mental health effects of limiting care during this pandemic, and potentially in future crises, on both cancer specialists and patients, who are used to unlimited resources for health care, may be far reaching. Having consensus guidelines to guide fair decision-making and developing empathic communication with regard to these issues is important.[57] Education and shifts in mindsets to prioritize the maximum health benefit for the community over the individual may be necessary in a country used to unlimited resources. Guidelines have been developed for low resource communities that may prove useful.[58,59]

It is unclear what effects these COVID-19 provoked changes in cancer screening and management will have on long-term cancer outcomes. In the United States, an estimated additional 87,001 deaths occurred in March and most of April 2020 compared with the last 6 years, of which 35% (30,755) were not directly attributable to COVID-19 (and in 14 states, >50% of excess deaths frame were not attributable).[60] Almost half (48%) of US people surveyed had a family member who had delayed medical care during the pandemic, with 10% stating that that member's medical condition worsened during the delay.[61] One modeling study of 6281 new stage 1 to 3 cancer cases in the United Kingdom who were delayed multidisciplinary workup during the pandemic suggested that an additional 181 lives and 3316 life years would be lost with a conservative estimate of only 25% of cases backlogged for 2 months.[62]

During the early phases of the pandemic, the number of new cancers diagnosed decreased.[63,64] This drop was likely secondary to patients not presenting for care and not a true drop in incidence. Thus, these cancers will come to the radar eventually at a greater size or stage than they would have with earlier detection, which may affect prognosis. A model that assumed only a 6-month disruption of care during the pandemic estimated the potential excess deaths from breast and colorectal cancer secondary to the pandemic disruptions in care demonstrates an excess of more than 10,000 deaths in the next decade, peaking in the first few years.[65] This model does not account for the increased morbidity, with possible more extensive surgeries including more mastectomies or more need for chemotherapy secondary to later presentations of disease.

Previous studies have demonstrated worsened outcomes during economic downturns, and in times of stress, and so it is likely the effects on breast cancer detection and management combined with the economic and societal effects of the pandemic will lead to effects on long-term outcomes.[66] It is also plausible that if there are not measurable deleterious effects from these delays, then reimbursements for care may be renegotiated or guidelines may shift to reduce care.

EFFECTS ON HOSPITALS AND RADIOLOGISTS OF CHANGES IN CARE

The COVID-19 pandemic has had marked economic effects on the health care system, academic radiology departments, and radiology practices. A survey conducted by ACR and the Radiology Business Management Association reported that 97.4% of 228 radiology practices (urban, academic, and rural) experienced declines in imaging volume in March/April 2020, with a drop of greater than 90% of elective procedures and 60% of urgent procedures.[13] One-third of academic radiology chairs reported a near two-thirds decrease in volume with some reporting an 80% drop in hard hit areas.[34] Greater than 82% of chairs had at least a 50% decrease in total radiology volume at the nadir.[34]

Breast imaging was disproportionately affected by postponed cases. The largest health care system in New York reported a drop of 88% affecting all modality types, with mammography use plummeting by 94%, MR imaging 74%, and ultrasound 64%.[67] In another study of 6 academic medical centers across the United States, 3 centers in regions with lower rates of COVID-19, radiology volumes declined steeply from calendar week 11 to 16 with a range of 40% to 70% total volume drop at the lowest drop.[68] Of those drops, screening mammography was among the most significant drop, as well as slowest in recovering. The reduction in screening mammography went as far as 99% in weeks 15 and 16. Diagnostic mammography volumes did not drop as dramatically, however still hit a low of 85% volume decrease at the nadir in week 16.[68]

On gradual reopenings of care (in May–July in most centers), a significant backlog of past studies had built. In addition, significant changes in scheduling with increased evening or weekend hours, changes in protocols for shorter MR imaging scan times,[68] and off-loading studies from hospitals and cancer centers to protect higher risk patients were required to allow for more spacing. Changes to patient registration and check-in, pre-screening for symptoms, PPE requirements, and disinfection protocols were instituted briskly. One hundred percent of academic radiology departments reported reorganizing the waiting rooms and dressing areas to comply with social distancing mandates.[34]

Radiology practices restructured reading rooms and implemented home PACS. Some practices shifted rapidly to home PACS, moving from 100% of radiologists onsite to 80% reading from home within a few weeks.[69] However, for breast imaging, this process is more complicated and expensive due to quality compliance requirements, the need for high-resolution monitors, and the need to be on site for diagnostic and interventions and happened at much lower levels. Telehealth increased in general, for patient surgery, oncology, and genetics appointments, as well as for virtual multidisciplinary tumor boards, leading to fewer in person multidisciplinary consults. Educational conferences and lectures moved to virtual platforms such as Webex, Microsoft Teams, and Zoom.[13,70] The effect of increased telecommuting and telehealth remain unclear. Telecommuting may increase radiologist morale, flexibility, and even potentially productivity, or alternatively it may decrease collaborations, interfacing with multidisciplinary colleagues, educational value, or productivity.[71] About half of the radiologists surveyed nationwide believed that teleradiology would continue and lead to increased efficiency.[13]

The marked reductions in volume have devastating financial implications to practices. Half of the health care practices in California furloughed or laid off employees and almost two-thirds reduced staff hours.[61,72] In academic practices, a quarter had furloughed or laid off staff.[34] Significant reductions in radiologist and staff incomes (in about 50% of practices in one survey), personal and academic protected time, research endeavors, workload, hours, professional funds, bonuses and financial incentives, and retirement allocations occurred amid hiring freezes and workspaces changes.[13] In a survey of 228 practices from across the country, there were mean reductions in both receipts and gross charges on average about 50%,[13] and greater than 70% of respondents reported applying for some sort of governmental financial relief. Although emergency governmental funds for financial relief were dispensed to hospitals and health care organizations through The Coronavirus Aid, Relief, and Economic Security Act and the Paycheck Protection Program and Health Care Enhancement Act (on the order of nearly $200 billion dollars), these funds are likely not enough to prevent lasting financial implications from the significant disruptions in volume and care.[73,74] Although practices are recovering, some near fully, as of September 2020, the anticipated time to full recovery remains unknown.

Effects on radiologist's mental health through this crisis have been significant. More than 60% of 600 radiologists in 44 states rated their anxiety as a 7 out of 10 during the pandemic.[75] In addition to having work and economic worries, some radiologists and staff were redeployed in the early days in hotspots to better serve COVID-19 patient care. In addition, many radiologists have had increased burdens at home with unexpected need to provide childcare and teaching duties for virtual schooling amid school and childcare care closures.[76] In addition, more than one-third of radiologists thought that they did not have adequate teleradiology capabilities during the pandemic, and about half said they did not have adequate PPE for themselves or their patients.[75] Mental stress regarding personal and family health, disruptions to travel and schedule, and family members with lost jobs or decreased income also affects the potential for long-term burnout in radiologists to increase, and mitigation strategies for burnout should be used.[77]

DELAYS IN CLINICAL RESEARCH EDUCATION AND ACADEMIC MEETINGS

Radiology education has also been significantly disrupted during the COVID-19 pandemic, including the need for redeployment, changes to reading rooms and social distancing, and cessation of in person conferences and didactic learning.[78] Some radiologists, especially residents early in training, were redeployed to other areas, particularly hard-hit urban environments such as New York and Boston, with some medical students even graduating early to join the front lines in caring for COVID-19–infected patients. Approximately 40% of radiologists in one survey thought that the shift to socially distant interpretations and conferences had a deleterious effect on resident and fellow education.[13]

Hundreds of scientific and medical conferences including dozens of radiology conferences were canceled or moved to virtual formats.[79] Significant impacts on networking, collaboration, committee work, vendor marketing, scientific presentations, and sharing of research are likely that may affect scientific progress as well as career choices.[80] Many radiologists were placed on institutional or state travel bans. Virtual grand rounds and virtual interviews both for education and for hiring were implemented during the pandemic. The cost and time savings of such virtual practices may prove to be practice changing after the pandemic is over.

Initially, most academic centers and universities suspended research, especially all trials involving patients or in-person interactions.[81] Guidance on how best to preserve clinical trials, and maintain integrity for those interrupted, was offered by the senior editorial staff at JAMA.[82] The FDA offered direction for those trials that may be disrupted.[83] Additional suggestions on how to avoid overestimation of disease-free survival if patients skip assessments and to report results from data during the pandemic separately from date before the pandemic continue to be offered.[82,83] In contrast, the National Cancer Institute intentionally kept functioning at 100% and stressed the importance of maintaining research to allow patients to have access to clinical trials and to maintain scientific progress, as well as to study the effects of COVID-19 in patients with cancer.[84] The National Cancer Institute (NCI) showed increased flexibility for prior minor infractions (such tests as a missed blood draw), recognizing that they may be necessary during COVID-19 to help maintain social distancing best practices for the patient. Some of the flexibility extended to clinical trials during the pandemic such as virtual, instead of in-person, visits for enrollment or assessments, the ability to receive tests and laboratory draws at sites closer to the patient that are not part of the trial sites, and decreases in the administrative tasks required prepandemic may carry over to the postpandemic world, perhaps making clinical trials more accessible to the general population.[85]

Of note, the pandemic led to the creation of unique opportunities for the creation of collaborative, crowdsourced research endeavors and databases, including the COVID-19 and Cancer Consortium, among others, collecting real-time data for observational trials.[86]

LONG-TERM RAMIFICATIONS AND REBUILDING

The final economic costs of the pandemic on the health care industry will likely be colossal. One study proposes the direct medical costs will approach $165 billion dollars if only 20% of the population is infected (53.8 million symptomatic cases) and would continue to cost up to a total of almost $215 billion in indirect costs in the year after discharge.[87] This figure will increase if the percent infected increased greater than that. Nationally, there has been significant deleterious effects on the economy including almost 17 million Americans filing for unemployment in a 3-week period over March/April alone, although with claims decreasing continually since that peak.[88,89] Whether or not COVID-19 will continue

to circulate in the population with annual or seasonal outbreaks or whether this will be an outbreak that has mostly cycled through the population with a return to closer to normal by 2022 or so remains unclear and debated yet at the time of this writing.

What is clear is that without a vaccine and other treatments, social distancing and PPE with masks and other protections for HCWs are likely to remain the primary weapons against the virus and will likely continue to play a part in daily life and in radiology practices and patient care in breast imaging centers for a while yet to come. What the future looks like on the other side of the pandemic remains unclear but will involve significant effects on both COVID-19– and non-COVID-19–related health outcomes, mental health outcomes, the national and global economy, radiology practices and breast centers, and on cancer outcomes, screening rates, and cancer management and treatment protocols.

CLINICS CARE POINTS

- If care is taken for protective measures for the patients and HCWs as outlined in different care algorithms, breast cancer treatment should continue during the pandemic, especially in light of the unknown timeframe of the crisis.
- It is unclear what effects these COVID-19 provoked changes in cancer screening and management will have on long term cancer outcomes.
- Radiology volumes dropped drastically during the early weeks of the pandemic, with the most dramatic reductions in screening mammography which came to a near complete halt for a few weeks in most places.
- Mental stress and workload changes increase the potential for long term burnout in radiologists to increase and mitigation strategies for burnout should be employed.

REFERENCES

1. Holshue ML, DeBolt C, Lindquist S, et al. First Case of 2019 Novel Coronavirus in the United States. N Engl J Med 2020;382:929–36.
2. Coronavirus Resource Center. Johns Hopkins University School of Medicine. Available at: https://coronavirus.jhu.edu. Accessed September 10, 2020.
3. World Health Organization. Responding to community spread of COVID-19: interim guidance, 7 March 2020. World Health Organization. Available at: https://apps.who.int/iris/handle/10665/331421. Accessed September 10, 2020.

4. Framework for Healthcare Systems Providing Non-COVID-19 Clinical Care During the COVID-19 Pandemic. Available at: https://www.cdc.gov/coronavirus/2019-ncov/hcp/framework-non-COVID-care.html. Updated June 30th. Accessed September 10, 2020.

5. Moy L, Toth HK, Newell MS, et al. Response to COVID-19 in Breast Imaging. J Breast Imaging 2020;2(3):180–5.

6. Sharpe RE Jr, Kuszyk BS, Mossa-Basha M, For the RSNA COVID-19 Task Force. Special Report of the RSNA COVID-19 Task Force: The Short- and Long-Term Financial Impact of the COVID-19 Pandemic on Private Radiology Practices. Radiology 2020. https://doi.org/10.1148/radiol.2020202517.

7. The coronavirus claims two Georgia health care workers. 2020. Available at: https://www.ajc.com/news/virus-claims-two-georgia-healthcare-workers/XTijtgzE6z2gcoZ7QLvPZN/. Accessed September 8, 2020.

8. Nguyen LH, Drew DA, Graham MS, et al. Risk of COVID-19 among front-line health-care workers and the general community: a prospective cohort study. Lancet Public Health 2020;5: e475–83.

9. Cinar P, Kubal T, Freifeld A, et al. Safety at the Time of the COVID-19 Pandemic: How to Keep our Oncology Patients and Healthcare Workers Safe. J Natl Compr Canc Netw 2020;1–6. https://doi.org/10.6004/jnccn.2020.7572.

10. Lu M. The front line: visualizing the occupations with the highest COVID-19 risk. 2020. Available at: https://www.visualcapitalist.com/the-front-line-visualizing-the-occupations-with-the-highest-COVID-19-risk/. Accessed September 9, 2020.

11. ASBrS and ACR Joint Statement on Breast Screening Exams During the COVID-19 Pandemic. 2020. Available at: https://www.sbi-online.org/Portals/0/Position%20Statements/2020/society-of-breast-imaging-statement-on-breast-imaging-during-COVID19-pandemic.pdf. Accessed September 9, 2020.

12. Society of Breast Imaging Statement on Breast Imaging during the COVID-19 Pandemic. 2020. Available at: https://www.sbi-online.org/Portals/0/Position%20Statements/2020/society-of-breast-imaging-statement-on-breast-imaging-during-COVID19-pandemic.pdf. Accessed September 9, 2020.

13. Malhotra A, Wu X, Fleishon HB, et al. Initial Impact of Coronavirus Disease 2019 (COVID-19) on Radiology Practices: An ACR/RBMA Survey [published online ahead of print, 2020 Aug 4]. J Am Coll Radiol 2020. https://doi.org/10.1016/j.jacr.2020.07.028.

14. Canadian Society of Breast Imaging and Canadian Association of Radiologists Joint Position Statement on COVID-19. 2020. Available at: https://csbi.ca/wp-content/uploads/2020/03/Covid-19-statement-CSBI_CAR-1.pdf. Accessed. September 14, 2020.

15. Society of Breast Imaging Statement on Screening in a Time of Social Distancing. 2020. Available at: https://www.sbi-online.org/Portals/0/Position%20Statements/2020/SBI-statement-on-screening-in-a-time-of-social-distancing_March-17-2020.pdf. Accessed September 10, 2020.

16. Pediconi F, Mann RM, Gilbert FJ, et al. on behalf of the EUSOBI Executive Board. EUSOBI recommendations for breast imaging and cancer diagnosis during and after the COVID-19 pandemic. 2020. Available at: https://www.eusobi.org/content-eusobi/uploads/EUSOBI-Recommendations_Breast-Imaging-during-COVID.pdf. Accessed September 9, 2020.

17. Pediconi F, Galati F, Bernardi D, et al. Breast imaging and cancer diagnosis during the COVID-19 pandemic: recommendations from the Italian College of Breast Radiologists by SIRM. Radiol Med 2020;125(10):926–30.

18. American College of Surgeons. COVID-19: Guidance for Triage of Non-Emergent Surgical Procedures. 2020. Available at: https://www.facs.org/covid-19/clinical-guidance/triage. Accessed September 10, 2020.

19. Bartlett DL, Howe JR, Chang G, et al. Management of Cancer Surgery Cases During the COVID-19 Pandemic: Considerations. Ann Surg Oncol 2020; 27:1717–20.

20. Soran A, Brufsky A, Gimbel M, et al. Breast Cancer Diagnosis, Treatment and Follow-Up During COVID-19 Pandemic. Eur J Breast Health 2020; 16(2):86–8.

21. Sheng JY, Santa-Maria CA, Mangini N, et al. Management of Breast Cancer During the COVID-19 Pandemic: A Stage- and Subtype-Specific Approach [published online ahead of print, 2020 Jun 30]. JCO Oncol Pract 2020. https://doi.org/10.1200/OP.20.00364.

22. Smith BL, Nguyen A, Korotkin JE, et al. A system for risk stratification and prioritization of breast cancer surgeries delayed by the COVID-19 pandemic: preparing for re-entry. Breast Cancer Res Treat 2020. https://doi.org/10.1007/s10549-020-05792-2.

23. Dietz JR, Moran MS, Isakoff SJ, et al. Recommendations for prioritization, treatment, and triage of breast cancer patients during the COVID-19 pandemic the COVID-19 pandemic breast cancer consortium. Breast Cancer Res Treat 2020. https://doi.org/10.1007/s10549-020-05644-z.

24. American College of Surgeons, American Society of Anesthesiologists. Association of periOperative Registered Nurses, American Hospital Association. Joint Statement: Roadmap for Resuming Elective Surgery after COVID-19 Pandemic. 2020. Available at: https://www.facs.org/covid-19/clinical-guidance/roadmap-elective-surgery. Accessed September 9, 2020.

25. Curigliano G, Banerjee S, Cervantes A, et al. Managing cancer patients during the COVID-19 pandemic: an ESMO multidisciplinary expert consensus [published online ahead of print, 2020 Jul 31]. Ann Oncol 2020. https://doi.org/10.1016/j.annonc.2020.07.010.

26. Hanna TP, Evans GA, Booth CM. Cancer, COVID-19 and the precautionary principle: prioritizing treatment during a global pandemic. Nat Rev Clin Oncol 2020;17:268–70.

27. Chan JJ, Sim Y, Ow SGW, et al. The impact of COVID-19 on and recommendations for breast cancer care: the Singapore experience. Endocr Relat Cancer 2020;27(9):R307–27.

28. Curigliano G, Cardoso MJ, Poortmans P, et al. Recommendations for triage, prioritization and treatment of breast cancer patients during the COVID-19 pandemic. Breast 2020;52:8–16.

29. de Azambuja E, Trapani D, Loibl S, et al. ESMO Management and treatment adapted recommendations in the COVID-19 era: Breast Cancer. ESMO Open 2020;5(Suppl 3):e000793.

30. ESMO. The ESMO-MCBS Score Card esmo.org. 2020. Available at: https://www.esmo.org/guidelines/esmo-mcbs/esmo-magnitude-of-clinical-benefit-scale. Accessed September 9, 2020.

31. ASCO Special Report: A Guide to Cancer Care Delivery During the COVID-19 Pandemic. 2020. Available at: https://www.asco.org/sites/new-www.asco.org/files/content-files/2020-ASCO-Guide-Cancer-COVID19.pdf. Accessed September 9, 2020.

32. ASCO Coronavirus Resources. Available at: https://www.asco.org/asco-coronavirus-information. Accessed September 10, 2020.

33. Spring LM, Specht MC, Jimenez RB, et al. Case 22-2020: A 62-Year-Old Woman with Early Breast Cancer during the Covid-19 Pandemic. N Engl J Med 2020;383(3):262–72.

34. Siegal DS, Wessman B, Zadorozny J, et al. Operational Radiology Recovery in Academic Radiology Departments After the COVID-19 Pandemic: Moving Toward Normalcy. J Am Coll Radiol 2020;17(9):1101–7.

35. ACR Response to COVID-19. 2020. Available at: https://accreditationsupport.acr.org/support/solutions/articles/11000084016-acr-response-to-covid-19-created-03-20-2020-?_ga=2.106697866.8219742 01.1585157241-178615201.1580929929. Accessed September 10, 2020.

36. Coronavirus (COVID-19) Update: FDA prepares for resumption of domestic inspections with new risk assessment system. 2020. Available at: https://www.fda.gov/news-events/press-announcements/coronavirus-covid-19-update-fda-prepares-resumption-domestic-inspections-new-risk-assessment-system. Accessed September 8, 2020.

37. Yu J, Ouyang W, Chua MLK, et al. SARS-CoV-2 Transmission in patients with cancer at a tertiary care hospital in Wuhan, China [published online March 25]. JAMA Oncol 2020. https://doi.org/10.1001/jamaoncol.2020.0980.

38. Liang W, Guan W, Chen R, et al. Cancer patients in SARS-CoV-2 infection: a nationwide analysis in China. Lancet Oncol 2020;21(3):335–7.

39. Zhang L, Zhu F, Xie L, et al. Clinical characteristics of COVID-19-infected cancer patients: a retrospective case study in three hospitals within Wuhan, China. Ann Oncol 2020;31(7):894–901.

40. Wu Z, McGoogan JM. Characteristics of and important lessons from the coronavirus disease 2019 (COVID-19) outbreak in China: Summary of a report of 72314 cases from the Chinese Center for Disease Control and Prevention. JAMA 2020;323(13):1239–42.

41. Mehta V, Goel S, Kabarriti R, et al. Case fatality rate of cancer patients with COVID-19 in a New York hospital system. Cancer Discov 2020. https://doi.org/10.1158/2159-8290.CD-20-0516.

42. Miyashita H, Mikami T, Chopra N, et al. Do patients with cancer have a poorer prognosis of COVID-19? An experience in New York City. Ann Oncol 2020. https://doi.org/10.1016/j.annonc.2020.04.006.

43. Kuderer NM, Choueiri TK, Shah DP, et al. Clinical impact of COVID-19 on patients with cancer (CCC19): a cohort study [published correction appears in Lancet. 2020;396(10253):758]. Lancet 2020;395(10241):1907–18.

44. Guan WJ, Ni ZY, Hu Y, et al. Clinical characteristics of coronavirus disease 2019 in China. N Engl J Med 2020;382:1708–20.

45. American Society of Clinical Oncology. ASCO Survey on COVID-19 in Oncology (ASCO) Registry. Available at: https://www.asco.org/asco-coronavirus-information/coronavirus-registry. Accessed September 10, 2020.

46. Lee LY, Cazier JB, Angelis V, et al. COVID-19 mortality in patients with cancer on chemotherapy or other anticancer treatments: a prospective cohort study [published correction appears in Lancet. 2020;396(10250):534]. Lancet 2020;395(10241):1919–26.

47. Printz C. When a global pandemic complicates cancer care: Although oncologists and their patients are accustomed to fighting tough battles against a lethal disease, Coronavirus Disease 2019 (COVID-19) has posed an unprecedented challenge. Cancer 2020;126(14):3171–3.

48. American College of Emergency Physicianns COVID-19. 2020. Available at: https://www.emergencyphysicians.org/globalassets/emphysicians/all-pdfs/acep-mc-COVID19-april-poll-analysis.pdf. Accessed September 8, 2020.

49. Vanni G, Materazzo M, Pellicciaro M, et al. Breast Cancer and COVID-19: The Effect of Fear on

Patients' Decision-making Process. In Vivo 2020; 34(3 Suppl):1651–9.

50. Papautsky EL, Hamlish T. Patient-reported treatment delays in breast cancer care during the COVID-19 pandemic. Breast Cancer Res Treat 2020. https://doi.org/10.1007/s10549-020-05828-7.

51. Medicare telemedicine health care provider fact sheet. 2020. Available at: https://www.cms.gov/newsroom/fact-sheets/medicare-telemedicine-health-care-provider-fact-sheet. Accessed September 8, 2020.

52. Yin K, Singh P, Drohan B, et al. Breast imaging, breast surgery, and cancer genetics in the age of COVID-19 [published online ahead of print, 2020 Aug 4]. Cancer 2020. https://doi.org/10.1002/cncr.33113.

53. Xie C, Wang X, Liu H, et al. Outcomes in Radiotherapy-Treated Patients With Cancer During the COVID-19 Outbreak in Wuhan, China [published online ahead of print, 2020 Jul 30]. JAMA Oncol 2020;e202783. https://doi.org/10.1001/jamaoncol.2020.2783.

54. de Joode K, Dumoulin DW, Engelen V, et al. Impact of the coronavirus disease 2019 pandemic on cancer treatment: the patients' perspective. Eur J Cancer 2020;136:132–9.

55. Gharzai LA, Resnicow K, An LC, et al. Perspectives on Oncology-Specific Language During the Coronavirus Disease 2019 Pandemic: A Qualitative Study [published online ahead of print, 2020 Aug 6]. JAMA Oncol 2020;e202980. https://doi.org/10.1001/jamaoncol.2020.2980.

56. Oncology Language for the COVID-19 Pandemic. 2020. Available at: https://www.nccn.org/covid-19/pdf/Oncology%20Langauge-Communicating%20Changes%20in%20Delivery%20of%20Care.pdf. Accessed September 8, 2020.

57. Emanuel EJ, Persad G, Upshur R, et al. Fair Allocation of Scarce Medical Resources in the Time of Covid-19. N Engl J Med 2020;382(21):2049–55.

58. DeBoer RJ, Fadelu TA, Shulman LN, et al. Applying Lessons Learned From Low-Resource Settings to Prioritize Cancer Care in a Pandemic. JAMA Oncol 2020;6(9):1429–33.

59. Yip CH, Anderson BO. The Breast Health Global Initiative: clinical practice guidelines for management of breast cancer in low- and middle-income countries. Expert Rev Anticancer Ther 2007;7(8):1095–104.

60. Woolf SH, Chapman DA, Sabo RT, et al. Excess Deaths From COVID-19 and Other Causes, March-April 2020. JAMA 2020;324(5):510–3.

61. Hamel L, Kearney A, Kirsinger A, et al. KFF Health Tracking Poll. 2020. Available at: https://www.kff.org/report-section/kff-health-tracking-poll-late-april-2020-economic-and-mental-health-impacts-of-coronavirus/. Accessed September 10, 2020.

62. Sud A, Torr B, Jones ME, et al. Effect of delays in the 2-week-wait cancer referral pathway during the COVID-19 pandemic on cancer survival in the UK: a modelling study. Lancet Oncol 2020. https://doi.org/10.1016/s1470-2045(20)30392-2.

63. IJzerman M, Emery J. Is a delayed cancer diagnosis a consequence of COVID-19?. 2020. Available at: https://pursuit.unimelb.edu.au/articles/is-a-delayed-cancer-diagnosis-a-consequence-of-covid-19. Accessed September 9, 2020.

64. Kaufman HW, Chen Z, Niles J, et al. Changes in the Number of US Patients With Newly Identified Cancer Before and During the Coronavirus Disease 2019 (COVID-19) Pandemic. JAMA Netw Open 2020; 3(8):e2017267.

65. Sharpless NE. COVID-19 and cancer. Science 2020; 368(6497):1290.

66. Maruthappu M, Watkins J, Noor AM, et al. Economic downturns, universal health coverage, and cancer mortality in high-income and middle-income countries, 1990-2010: a longitudinal analysis. Lancet 2016;388(10045):684–95.

67. Naidich JJ, Boltyenkov A, Wang JJ, et al. Impact of the Coronavirus Disease 2019 (COVID-19) Pandemic on Imaging Case Volumes. J Am Coll Radiol 2020;17(7):865–72.

68. Norbash AM, Moore AV Jr, Recht MP, et al. Early-Stage Radiology Volume Effects and Considerations with the Coronavirus Disease 2019 (COVID-19) Pandemic: Adaptations, Risks, and Lessons Learned. J Am Coll Radiol 2020;17(9):1086–95.

69. Sammer MBK, Sher AC, Huisman TAGM, et al. Response to the COVID-19 Pandemic: Practical Guide to Rapidly Deploying Home Workstations to Guarantee Radiology Services During Quarantine, Social Distancing, and Stay Home Orders [published online ahead of print, 2020 Jun 30]. AJR Am J Roentgenol 2020;1–4. https://doi.org/10.2214/AJR.20.23297.

70. Madox W. Coronavirus has sparked a teleradiology revolution. Available at: https://www.dmagazine.com/healthcare-business/2020/2004/coronavirus-has-sparked-a-teleradiology-revolution/. Accessed September 10, 2020.

71. Simons J. IBM, a pioneer of remote work, calls workers back to the office: Big Blue says move will improve collaboration and accelerate the pace of work. Wall St J 2017. Available at: https://www.wsj.com/articles/ibm-a-pioneer-of-remote-work-calls-workers-back-to-the-office-14 95108802. Accessed September 9, 2020.

72. Thousands of healthcare workers are laid off or furloughed as coronavirus spreads. Los Angeles Times 2020;. https://www.latimes.com/california/story/2020-05-02/coronavirus-california-healthcare-workers-layoffs-furloughs. Accessed September 8, 2020.

73. Coronavirus Aid, Relief, and Economic Security (CARES) Act. Pub L No 116-136 (2020).

74. Paycheck Protection Program and Health Care Enhancement Act. Pub L No 116-139 (2020).

75. Demirjian NL, Fields BKK, Song C, et al. Impacts of the Coronavirus Disease 2019 (COVID-19) pandemic on healthcare workers: A nationwide survey of United States radiologists. Clin Imaging 2020; 68:218–25.

76. Shanafelt T, Ripp J, Trockel M. Understanding and Addressing Sources of Anxiety Among Health Care Professionals During the COVID-19 Pandemic. JAMA 2020;323(21):2133–4.

77. Restauri N, Sheridan AD. Burnout and Posttraumatic Stress Disorder in the Coronavirus Disease 2019 (COVID-19) Pandemic: Intersection, Impact, and Interventions. J Am Coll Radiol 2020;17(7): 921–6.

78. Alvin MD, George E, Deng F, et al. The Impact of COVID-19 on Radiology Trainees. Radiology 2020; 296(2):246–8.

79. Kalia V, Srinivasan A, Wilkins L, et al. Adapting Scientific Conferences to the Realities Imposed by COVID-19. Radiol Imaging Cancer 2020;2(4): e204020.

80. Evens R. The impact of a pandemic on professional meetings. Radiol Imaging Cancer 2020;2(3). Available at: https://pubs.rsna.org/doi/10.1148/rycan.2020204012. Accessed October 2, 2020.

81. Vagal A, Reeder SB, Sodickson DK, et al. The Impact of the COVID-19 Pandemic on the Radiology Research Enterprise: Radiology Scientific Expert Panel. Radiology 2020;296(3):E134–40.

82. McDermott MM, Newman AB. Preserving clinical trial integrity during the coronavirus pandemic. JAMA 2020. https://doi.org/10.1001/jama.2020.4689.

83. FDA guidance on conduct of clinical trials of medical products during COVID-19 pandemic: guidance for industry, investigators, and institutional review boards. US Food and Drug Administration. 2020. Available at: https://www.fda.gov/media/136238/download. Accessed September 11, 2020.

84. Eary J, Shankar L. COVID-19 Update from the NCI Cancer Imaging Program. Radiol Imaging Cancer 2020;2(3):e204017.

85. Nabhan C, Choueiri TK, Mato AR. Rethinking Clinical Trials Reform During the COVID-19 Pandemic. JAMA Oncol 2020;6(9):1327–9.

86. COVID-19 and Cancer Consortium Registry (CCC19). ClinicalTrials.gov identifier: NCT04354701. 2020. Available at: https://www.clinicaltrials.gov/ct2/show/NCT04354701?term=NCT04354701&draw=2&rank=1. Accessed September 11, 2020.

87. Bartsch SM, Ferguson MC, McKinnell JA, et al. The Potential Health Care Costs And Resource Use Associated With COVID-19 In The United States. Health Aff (Millwood) 2020;39(6):927–35.

88. Department of Labor. 2020. Available at: https://www.dol.gov/ui/data.pdf. Accessed September 10, 2020.

89. Cavallo JJ, Forman HP. The Economic Impact of the COVID-19 Pandemic on Radiology Practices. Radiology 2020;296(3):E141–4.

Breast Radiology Advocacy
Responding to the Call-to-Action

Amy K. Patel, MD*

KEYWORDS

- Radiology • Advocacy • Breast cancer • Mammography screening • Social media

KEY POINTS

- In an increasingly competitive and passionate health care environment, radiology advocacy is imperative, now more than ever.
- Advocacy and responding to the call-to-action are imperative for breast cancer patients to ensure access-to-care, education, and research funding.
- Social media has become a transformative avenue to disseminate widespread messaging at a rapid rate to breast cancer community stakeholders, particularly when it comes to screening mammography access.

INTRODUCTION

In an increasingly competitive and passionate health care environment, radiology political advocacy is imperative, now more than ever. Arguably, it is particularly more crucial in the world of breast cancer, as we as a breast cancer community are tirelessly assembling to advocate for our patients on a variety of levels, whether it is including but not limited to, breast cancer screening, diagnosis and treatment, access-to-care, education, or research funding. As breast radiologists, it is no longer simply enough to clock in our normal work hours; we must ALL make a concerted effort to vociferously advocate for our patients and profession. We must be the voice for those who do not have one or for those whose voices get lost in the, at times, deafening noise. Luckily, there are many avenues in which this championing can be achieved. In addition, the importance of radiology advocacy is being instilled in a new generation of radiologists at an unprecedented rate, largely in part to the exposure they are receiving to this facet of medicine very early in their training. Recognizing the importance of actively championing for our subspecialty and our patients is arguably just as important as one's clinical proficiency when entering practice. We must encourage the next generation to embrace this movement for change as we continue to face a perpetually changing and uncertain health care horizon.

BRIEF HISTORY OF RADIOLOGY POLITICAL ADVOCACY

There has been a long and rich history of political advocacy in health care, and particularly in radiology. "Advocate" comes from the Latin "ad" and "Vocare," to call. More current definitions of "Advocacy" revolve around efforts to affect some aspect of society, including individuals, employers, or the government.[1]

Oftentimes, "advocacy" and "lobbying" are used interchangeably. However, in both a regulatory and legal context, lobbying is advocacy that is focused on specific legislative pieces with clear reporting requirements and penalties for infractions.[1] Make no mistake: lobbying is crucial for access-to-care for our patients. The historical roots of lobbying date back to our founding fathers, with James Madison deeming a "faction" as "a number of citizens, whether amounting to a

Department of Radiology, University of Missouri-Kansas City School of Medicine, Liberty, MO, USA
* Liberty Hospital Women's Imaging, 2529 Glenn Hendren Drive, Suite G80, Liberty, MO 64068.
E-mail addresses: amykpatel64112@gmail.com; patelak@umkc.edu

Radiol Clin N Am 59 (2021) 13–17
https://doi.org/10.1016/j.rcl.2020.09.010
0033-8389/21/© 2020 Elsevier Inc. All rights reserved.

minority of the whole, who are united and actuated by some common impulse of passion, or of interest....”[2] However, the actual term "lobbyists" was first described during the time when President Ulysses S. Grant was in office and advocates would physically gather in the lobby of the Willard Hotel in Washington, DC, to gain access to him.[3] The health care industry accounts for approximately one-sixth of the US gross domestic product, so it is no surprise why the health care lobby is one of the most robust in Washington, DC.[1] Fortunately, radiology has arguably the most exemplary and knowledgeable governmental relations teams out of all medical subspecialties, serving as steadfast and effective lobbyists on behalf of our profession all year round. Together, our efforts supporting medical and radiology lobbying are crucial as we educate our elected officials, overseeing bodies, patients, and patient advocates.

ADVOCACY EDUCATION AT THE TRAINEE LEVEL

Radiology political advocacy is reaching our trainees and a new generation of radiologists at an unprecedented rate, largely in part to the exposure they are receiving to this facet of medicine very early in their training. In radiology, we have taken the term "advocacy" one step further to coin the term "radvocacy," a hybrid of "radiology" and "advocacy." In fact, this term was coined by a former trainee who is now a young radiologist, and spread via Twitter and social media. "Economics" is now one of the Accreditation Council for Graduate Medical Education milestones, and thus many residency programs are implementing advocacy curriculum, whether of their own or through other avenues such as the Radiology Leadership Institute.[4,5] This curriculum development, in and of itself, is inciting great enthusiasm and imparting essential knowledge to a new generation of future and early career radiologists who will hopefully carry the torch for years to come. In addition, comprehensive offerings in the form of fellowships have been established, including the American College of Radiology (ACR) Rutherford-Lavanty Fellowship in Government Relations. This fellowship was established in 1993 and was initially named the J.T. Rutherford Fellowship in honor of the first lobbyist of the ACR. It was renamed in 2014, adding Donald Lavanty's last name, an additional trailblazing ACR lobbyist with expertise in health care policy and law.[6,7] This fellowship exposes residents to the legislative and regulatory processes in which the ACR participates. It also exposes residents to how various governmental factors affect the future of radiology. Residents meet members of congress from both sides of the aisle, all of whom are in support of radiology legislative agendas such as screening mammography access. The overwhelming majority of trainees who experience this fellowship become ardent "radvocates" during their careers, largely in part to truly understanding the inner workings of how radiology's government relations team works tirelessly on behalf of our patients and profession.

EXAMPLES OF ADVOCACY AT THE LOCAL, STATE, AND NATIONAL LEVELS

The beauty of advocacy is that it can be expressed at so many levels and forms. Examples of local efforts include speaking or making your presence known at women's health events where you can empower women to make the best informed decisions for themselves (Fig. 1). At the institutional level, speaking to hospital systems at medical executive meetings and even meeting with referring providers and payers can be effective ways to advocate on behalf of our patients for the access and standard of care they deserve. Also, participating in podcasts can be a great way in which to disseminate messaging about screening mammography and access (https://www.acr.org/Practice-Management-Quality-Informatics/ACR-Bulletin/Podcasts/PHM-in-Your-Practice/PHM-and-Breast-Imaging).

Other ways include community involvement with organizations such as Susan G. Komen, American Cancer Society, Be Bright Pink, and The Pink Agenda. For example, through my involvement in Susan G. Komen Kansas and Western Missouri, I was named Komen's "Biggest Big Wig," a fundraising campaign in which I raised the most funds. From that endeavor, I was asked to throw the first pitch at the Kansas City Royals Major League Baseball Game. Before the first pitch, I was able to "make the pitch" of impressing on the fans the importance of annual screening mammography.

At the state level, you can get involved in your state radiological society. Each state has its own state radiological society that is a branch of the ACR.[8] Furthermore, you can be involved in legislative efforts, such as passing mammography legislation for digital breast tomosynthesis coverage, diagnostic breast imaging coverage, and supplemental screening. These efforts can be achieved by working with your state radiological society and respective lobbyist. The ACR's government relations staff can also be a great resource to assist in the initiation process. For example, through collaboration with the Missouri

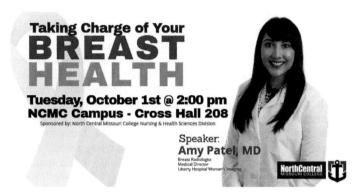

Fig. 1. Breast health advocacy poster. (*Courtesy of* North Central Missouri College, Trenton, MO; with permission.)

Radiological Society in 2018, we were able to pass critical legislation for digital breast tomosynthesis coverage for Missouri women annually beginning at age 40[9] (https://www.mycouriertribune.com/health/new-law-requires-insurance-to-cover-3d-mammograms-in-full-in-2019/article_259fb755-75cb-5574-b8e9-29c71e77e3a9.html#/questions/). More recently, I testified in front of the Missouri State Legislature with Senator Lauren Arthur (D) in support of Senate Bill 551, a bill that we crafted together, and was passed in August 2020, which will provide insurance coverage for high-risk breast cancer patients in accordance with the recommendations of the ACR/SBI screening recommendations in above average risk women (**Fig. 2**).

At the national level, involvement in the ACR and Radiology Advocacy Network (RAN) are at your disposal. In fact, one of the main pillars of the ACR is advocacy and health policy research, including placing emphasis on initiatives such as *Mammography Saves Lives* in collaboration with the SBI and the American Society of Breast Disease.[10]

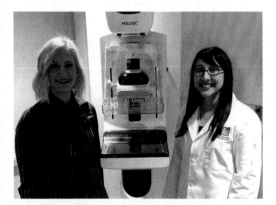

Fig. 2. The author and Senator Lauren Arthur in support of Senate Bill 551, a bill providing insurance coverage for high-risk breast cancer patients in accordance to the ACR/SBI screening recommendations in above average risk women.

The RAN is a grassroots advocacy network of the ACR that was devised to give states a voice, bringing them together in support of critical legislation and causes in the form of calls-to-action to relay our collective voices at the federal level.[11] The SBI is also another national organized radiology society in which to participate in advocacy efforts, with SBI having a robust Communications and Advocacy Task Force that also works tirelessly on behalf of our patients and the subspecialty of breast imaging.[12]

From a historical perspective, perhaps one of the most crowning achievements at the national level was the establishment of the Mammography Quality Standards Act (MQSA). This grassroots effort was initiated because many in the field of breast imaging felt that improvements were needed to standardize quality across the country, particularly regarding mammography imaging and dose. MQSA was then enacted by congress in 1992, requiring all mammography facilities to achieve minimum standards of quality for equipment, recordkeeping, and personnel. Implementing MQSA then fell under the jurisdiction of the Food and Drug Administration in 1993, and effective for mammography facilities to meet quality standards in 1994, including all US mammography facilities to become accredited by the ACR Mammography Accreditation Program.[13,14]

POLITICAL CONTRIBUTIONS AND ADVOCACY

Oftentimes, political contributions are not considered as a form of advocacy. However, they are just as, if not more, crucial as being a vocal advocate at any level. RADPAC, radiology's leading bipartisan political action committee, is instrumental in advocating on behalf of radiology specific legislation.[15] RADPAC has played an instrumental role in breast cancer screening legislation and access, with their efforts largely responsible for the extended moratorium of mammography screening in the reintroduction of the Protecting Access to Lifesaving Screenings (PALS) Act, cosponsored by ardent supporters of radiology legislation, Representative Debbie Wasserman Schultz (D) and Representative Susan W. Brooks (R).[16,17] At times, one may refer to this form of advocacy as "pay-to-play"; however, it remains the leading way for our voices to be heard, particularly at the federal level. At this level, the stakes are high, and every medical subspecialty is becoming increasingly competitive in this arena to make their voices heard and to protect their patients' interests.[16]

THE POWER OF BREAST CANCER SOCIAL MEDIA (#BCSM)

Social media has become a transformative avenue in which we disseminate messaging at such a rapid rate, even reaching populations historically difficult to access, including rural. The Centers for Disease Control and Prevention notes that "more than 100,000 lives could be saved each year if everyone in the United States received clinical preventive services," with cancer screening falling under this category.[18] As a result, social media is becoming increasingly relevant and important in today's society in how we vociferously advocate for causes and interact with our community members and the world. The unparalleled influence social media has on patients in relying on advice and education, for better or worse, makes this avenue crucial for us as a breast imaging community in which to participate. Using social media platforms, we can provide accurate information and advocate for initiatives such as mammography screening at rates of which we have never seen. In addition, it is an incredible way to reach a wide audience at the granular level, with certain platforms that can be used to target different demographics, particularly different patient ages. For example, Facebook has significantly increased involvement in health care initiatives, and in November 2019, established the "Facebook Preventive Health Tool" on its mobile app for US users to provide educational resources and up-

to-date recommendations.[19] Additional ways in which one can participate in advocacy efforts on social media include tweet chats, virtual journal clubs, Facebook live events, and conversations with certain factions on various social media platforms[20] (**Fig. 3**). Consequently, the hashtag "#BCSM", which stands for "breast cancer social media," is one of the most widely used and known breast cancer hashtags in the breast cancer social media community and is included in many social media posts, regardless of platform, so that up-to-date posts can be tracked regarding to the topic of breast cancer.[21] The more a hashtag is tracked, the more likely for widespread reach and dissemination of information.

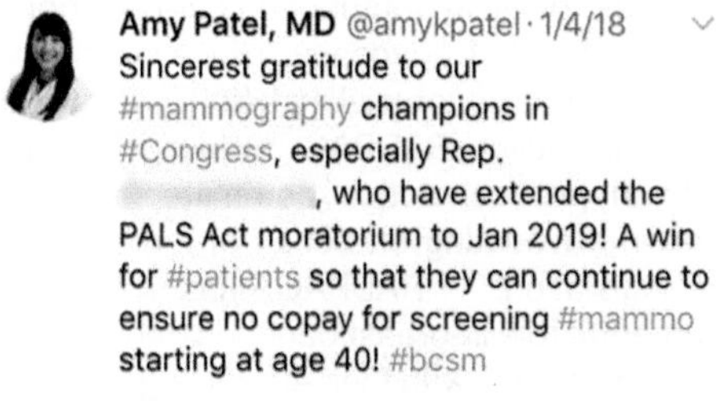

CALL-TO-ACTION

It has been incredible to see the call-to-action in our field in just a few years. We have been able to achieve so much; the moratorium to extend mammography screening at the federal level, the sweeping movement of breast imaging legislation being witnessed at the state level, and even local efforts, including patient and referring provider education and continuously advocating for our patients to have access to cutting edge technology, and simply, the standard of breast imaging care all patients deserve. I, myself, respond to the call-to-action every day, as for me, being a breast radiologist is not what I do; it's who I am. I fervently feel that we as a breast radiology community, must respond to the call-to-action; it is a moral imperative, and we owe it to the patients we serve. Often, my mammography technologists say they feel I inherently find more breast cancers because I am incredibly passionate about what I do. I challenge all to have that same passion for what we do as breast imagers and respond to the call-to-action beyond what we do in clinical practice. This moment in American history most certainly necessitates that, and we all, not just a select few, must be willing to rise to the occasion. Together as a breast imaging community, we are a formidable force, and our patients will be the victors in the end.

SUMMARY

The path of breast radiology advocacy has been paved by so many in our field; the breast imaging trailblazers, community organizers, steadfast patient advocates, and tireless lobbyists. Now, it is up to us to respond to the call-to-action. As health care becomes increasingly competitive, it will require persistent and deliberate efforts to remain at the forefront of what our patients require and

Amy Patel, MD @amykpatel · 1/4/18
Sincerest gratitude to our #mammography champions in #Congress, especially Rep. ▨▨▨▨▨▨▨, who have extended the PALS Act moratorium to Jan 2019! A win for #patients so that they can continue to ensure no copay for screening #mammo starting at age 40! #bcsm

Fig. 3. Social media tweet.

deserve. As Dr Zeke Silva, former Chair of the ACR Economics Commission once wrote, "Make Advocacy Automatic."[22] Together, we can continue to move the needle forward so we can ensure access to lifesaving tools such as testing and treatment so that ultimately, we achieve our paramount goal: to save the most lives and life years saved.

DISCLOSURE

A.K. Patel has no relevant commercial or financial conflicts of interest.

REFERENCES

1. Fleishon H. Advocacy in Radiology. J Am Coll Radiol 2014;11(8):751–3.
2. Hamilton A, Madison J, Jay J. The Federalist Project. The Federalist Papers. Available at: https://www.thefederalistpapers.org/wp-content/uploads/2012/12/The-Complete-Federalist-Papers.pdf. Accessed May 30, 2020.
3. The origins of 'lobbyist'. From the front hallways to the back rooms. Available at: https://www.merriam-webster.com/words-at-play/the-origins-of-lobbyist. Accessed May 28, 2020.
4. Prober A, Ledermann E, Norbash A, et al. Fulfilling the health care economics milestones: adopting an online curriculum for radiology residency programs. J Am Coll Radiol 2015;12(3):314–7.
5. RLI Resident Milestones Program. Economics and the physician's role in health care systems. Available at: https://www.acr.org/Practice-Management-Quality-Informatics/Radiology-Leadership-Institute/Programs-and-Training/RLI-Resident-Milestones-Program. Accessed May 30, 2020.
6. Rutherford-Lavanty fellowship in government relations. Available at: https://www.acr.org/Member-Resources/rfs/fellowships/Rutherford-Lavanty-Fellowship. Accessed May 30, 2020.
7. Lavanty D. Available at: https://www.marymount.edu/Home/Contact-Us/Faculty-Staff-Directory?lang=en-US&profileid=2146&page=5. Accessed May 30, 2020.
8. Benefits of the ACR and its state chapters. Available at: https://www.acr.org/Member-Resources/ACR-Chapters/Chapter-Benefits. Accessed May 27, 2020.
9. Missouri secures tomosynthesis coverage. Available at: https://www.acr.org/Advocacy-and-Economics/Advocacy-News/Advocacy-News-Issues/In-the-June-9-2018-Issue/Missouri-Secures-Tomosynthesis-Coverage. Accessed May 20, 2020.
10. ACR Fact Sheet. Available at: https://www.acr.org/About-ACR/Fact-Sheet. Accessed May 30, 2020.
11. Radiology Advocacy Network. Available at: https://cqrcengage.com/acradiology/home?0. Accessed May 30, 2020.
12. Society of Breast Imaging. Committees. Available at: https://www.sbi-online.org/ABOUTSBI/Committees.aspx#:~:text=The%20Task%20Force%20is%20a,areas%20of%20communications%20and%20advocacy.&text=*Must%20be%20a%20Fellow%20of%20SBI%20(FSBI)%20to%20apply. Accessed May 20, 2020.
13. Reynolds H. The big squeeze: a social and political history of the controversial mammogram. Ithaca (NY): Cornell University Press; 2012.
14. Destouet JM, Bassett LW, Yaffe MJ, et al. The ACR's mammography accreditation program: ten years of experience since MQSA. J Am Coll Radiol 2005; 2(7):585–94.
15. RADPAC. Available at: https://www.radpac.org/Login?returnUrl=%2f. Accessed May 20, 2020.
16. Patel AK, Balthazar P, Rosenkrantz A, et al. Characteristics of federal political contributions of self-identified radiologists across the United States. J Am Coll Radiol 2018;15(8):1068–72.
17. Press Release. Reps. Wasserman Schultz and Brooks reintroduce legislation to protect women's access to mammograms. Available at: https://wassermanschultz.house.gov/news/documentsingle.aspx?DocumentID=2343. Accessed May 29, 2020.
18. Merchant R. Evaluating the potential role of social media in preventive health care. JAMA 2020;323(5).
19. Facebook. Preventive Health. Available at: https://preventivehealth.facebook.com/. Accessed May 25, 2020.
20. Slanetz P, Patel AK, Sun MR, et al. Radiology advocacy-the time has come! J Am Coll Radiol 2019;16(11):1595–7.
21. Breast Cancer Social Media. Breast cancer hashtags. Available at: https://www.symplur.com/topic/breast-cancer/. Accessed May 30, 2020.
22. Silva Z. Make advocacy automatic. J Am Coll Radiol 2010;8(3):157–8.

Overdiagnosis and Risks of Breast Cancer Screening

Colleen H. Neal, MD*, Mark A. Helvie, MD[1]

KEYWORDS

• Overdiagnosis • Screening • Mammography • Breast cancer • Risks • Harms

KEY POINTS

- The benefits of screening mammography include early diagnosis, reduced breast cancer-associated mortality, and reduced treatment-associated morbidity.
- The risks of screening mammography include overdiagnosis/overtreatment, false-positive screening, false-positive biopsy, and radiation exposure.
- Overdiagnosis of breast cancer is a consequence of screening, and is more common in older women. When lead time and background incidence of breast cancer are adjusted for, the most reliable estimates of breast cancer overdiagnosis are less than 10%.
- For most women 40 years of age and over, the potential benefit of breast cancer screening outweighs its risks.

INTRODUCTION

Breast cancer remains a substantial health risk for women worldwide. In 2020, the American Cancer Society estimates that 276,480 women in the United States will be diagnosed with invasive breast cancer, and over 42,000 women will die.[1] Despite this sobering statistic, the mortality would be higher if not for the widespread implementation of screening mammography in the United States 3 decades ago. Since its introduction, screening mammography has contributed to a 40% reduction in breast cancer associated mortality among US women from 1989 to 2016.[2] Using Cancer Intervention and Surveillance Modeling Network (CISNET) data, Plevritis and colleagues[3] reported a 49% reduction in breast cancer-associated mortality from 2000 to 2012 because of screening mammography and therapeutic advances. Helvie and colleagues[4] reported a 37% decrease in late-stage disease from 2007 to 2009, compared with the prescreening era. Depending on the background incidence rate of breast cancer used in the modeling, Hendrick and colleagues[5] estimated that 384,046 to 614,484 breast cancer deaths have been averted since 1989, because of screening and treatment advances. Tabar and colleagues[6] evaluated long-term Swedish data and found that women who participated in organized breast cancer screening had a 60% lower risk of dying from breast cancer within 10 years after diagnosis and a 47% lower risk of dying 20 years after diagnosis compared with nonscreened participants with access to comparable stage-specific national treatment protocols. These results demonstrated that women who have participated in screening mammography obtain a significantly greater benefit from available therapies at the time of diagnosis than do those who have not participated. Overall, screening mammography has contributed considerably to the health of women in the United States over

Department of Radiology, Breast Imaging Division, University of Michigan, Ann Arbor, MI, USA
[1] Present address: 2910N TC SPC 5326, 1500 East Medical Center Drive, Ann Arbor, MI 48109.
* Corresponding author. Department of Radiology, University of Michigan, C415 MIB SPC 5842, 1500 East, Medical Center Drive, Ann Arbor, MI 48109.
E-mail address: hawleyc@med.umich.edu

Radiol Clin N Am 59 (2021) 19–27
https://doi.org/10.1016/j.rcl.2020.09.005
0033-8389/21/© 2020 Elsevier Inc. All rights reserved.

the last 30 years. However, like all medical tests and procedures, screening mammography is imperfect and has associated risks. These risks include overdiagnosis and overtreatment, false-positive examinations, and radiation exposure. In order to make the most appropriate care decisions for themselves, patients should be aware of the benefits and risks of screening mammography.

OVERDIAGNOSIS
Definition

Overdiagnosis is the concept that breast cancer detected at screening may not become clinically apparent or harm a patient in her lifetime. Overdiagnosis is often cited among the most harmful risks of breast cancer screening[7,8], due to the ensuing treatment (overtreatment) that may cause physical and/or psychosocial morbidity. Overdiagnosis can be conceptualized as 2 types. Type I overdiagnosis, which has also been referred to as obligate overdiagnosis,[9] is a screen-detected cancer that would not have become clinically evident prior to a patient's death from a noncancer etiology, such as cardiovascular disease. If the patient's death occurs during the mammographic lead time, caused by something other than breast cancer, it represents an example of Type I overdiagnosis. Because women of more advanced age have higher competing causes of mortality, the risk of Type I overdiagnosis is higher for older women. Type II overdiagnosis, which has been referred to as nonobligate overdiagnosis, is a screen-detected breast cancer that is extremely indolent (nonobligate progression) or possibly may even regress. However, breast cancer regression is extremely low in likelihood. In 2017, an expert group of radiologists who had interpreted a total of 6.8 million screening mammograms and diagnosed over 34,000 breast cancers reported zero cases of breast cancer regression out of 479 untreated, screen-detected invasive and noninvasive breast cancers.[10] Indolent, nonprogressive breast cancer is possible, particularly in older, postmenopausal women. However, the genetic events associated with breast cancer progression are not yet fully understood. Thus, it is not currently possible to discern which breast cancers will remain indolent. As scientific knowledge of breast cancer genetics and tailored therapies improves, science may be able to prospectively identify biologically indolent tumors and allow for limited or no treatment in some cases. This will reduce the individual risks of overdiagnosis and associated overtreatment.

Measuring Overdiagnosis

The incidence of overdiagnosed breast cancer is not quantifiable as an absolute number, and attempts to estimate overdiagnosis are complicated. The lack of a standardized method to measure breast cancer overdiagnosis is readily evident in the wide array of published estimates, ranging from 1% to 57%.[11-13] A direct quantification would require following a large cohort of women with similar breast cancer risk and untreated screen-detected breast cancers over an extended period of time, and then measuring the percentage of breast cancers that do not manifest clinically.[11] Such a study is not ethically feasible because of the possible harm it may cause patients. Furthermore, few women would willingly forgo treatment, leading to a small study cohort that could not be used to inform treatment for a large population of women. Therefore, overdiagnosis measurements are often estimated from randomized control trial (RCT) and observational study data as the difference between the observed and expected (absent screening) breast cancer incidence. There is large discrepancy among published overdiagnosis estimates, in part secondary to disputes over the expected incidence. One method to quantify overdiagnosis is outlined as follows. It starts with the observation of cumulative breast cancer incidence during and following a screening RCT. During the intervention portion of the trial, breast cancer incidence in the screening arm would be greater than the control group, because diagnoses are brought forward chronologically earlier. At the completion of the RCT, breast cancer incidences in the control and study patients then are observed over an extended period of time (equal to or greater than the mammographic lead time distribution) with neither arm participating in any additional screening. In randomized groups of equal-risk patients, the cumulative breast cancer incidence should be the same in both groups over time if there is no overdiagnosis. An extended observation period of at least 10 years[14] would be necessary to allow control patients to reach the incidence of the patients invited to screen. However, this type of observation from an RCT is often not possible, because multiple RCTs invited the control group to screen at the completion of the trial, rendering an overdiagnosis estimate unreliable.

The Malmö trial did not invite the control group to screen after completion of the trial, and thus may provide the best opportunity to quantify overdiagnosis. Inviting women age 55 to 69 (at randomization) to screening detected 10% more breast cancers (invasive and noninvasive) than became clinically evident in age-matched control subjects at 15 years of follow-up.[15] When noninvasive breast cancers were excluded, an overdiagnosis rate of 7% was estimated. It has been postulated that if members of the screening arm continued screening after the trial,[16,17] then the observed incidence of breast cancer in the screened patients would increase, thus increasing the overdiagnosis estimate, with a potential of 10% as the maximum overdiagnosis estimated as the result of mammographic screening.[16] Conversely, a fraction of control patients (25% in the Malmö and Canadian trials) reported opportunistic screening in the trial and follow-up period, which may have led to an underestimate of overdiagnosis.[18]

The Canadian National Breast Screening Studies (CNBSS-1 and CNBSS-2) were RCTs that did not systematically invite the control patients to screen at the close of the trial. In 2016, Baines and colleagues[19] evaluated the data from the CNBSS trials, and reported that 20 years after cessation of screening, overdiagnosis of invasive breast cancer was 48% for CNBSS-1 (women 40–49 years of age) and 5% for CNBSS-2 (women 50–59 years of age). However, when Marmot and colleagues[18] analyzed the CNBSS trial data, they reported an overdiagnosis estimate of 12.4% and 9.7% for CNBSS-1 and 2 respectively. The marked difference between these 2 authors' overdiagnosis estimates may be explained by the denominators used in the overdiagnosis calculations. For example, the estimate by Marmot and colleagues varied whether the denominator used was the "cancers diagnosed over the entire follow-up period" or the "cancers diagnosed during the screening period." The denominator in the latter example is lower, leading to a higher estimate of overdiagnosis. When overdiagnosis rates from the Malmö and both Canadian RCTs were calculated using variable denominators, the estimates ranged from 9.7% to 29.4%.[18] The denominator used in the overdiagnosis calculation may depend on the purpose of the estimate. For example, if the calculation is being made from a population perspective, a denominator that includes all breast cancers diagnosed in women of all ages would be used, whereas if the purpose is to calculate from an individual patient's risk of being overdiagnosed, a denominator that includes women of screening age and older may be used.[20] When the aggregate RCT data were calculated from a population perspective, Marmot and colleagues[18] estimated an 11% risk of overdiagnosis. Similarly, de Gelder and colleagues[20] demonstrated the extent to which overdiagnosis estimates are influenced by the denominator used.

Working with observational incidence data from the Dutch screening program from 1990 to 2006, her group found that the estimated overdiagnosis rate could vary by a factor of 3.5 when different denominators were used.

The Swedish Two-County and Gothenburg trials are examples where the control group was offered screening at the completion of the study arm. 6 to 8 years after randomization, the control group was invited to screening. Yen and colleagues[17] note that in the Swedish Two-County trial, the "catch-up" of the control group's breast cancer incidence began immediately after they were invited to screen, indicating that any degree of overdiagnosis is largely incurred at the prevalence screen. At 29 years of follow-up, Yen reported no excess incidence of breast cancer in the patients invited to screen in the Swedish Two-County Trial, whether or not in situ disease is included (relative risk [RR] 1.00, confidence interval [CI] 0.92-1.08). Evaluating the data by patient age at randomization, no excess cancer incidence was seen in any of the active study cohorts except the oldest (aged 70–74 years of age at randomization), although this was nonsignificant (RR 1.25, CI 0.97–1.61). In this age group, a higher degree of overdiagnosis may be expected because of the higher competing mortality causes. Overall, long-term follow-up data from the Two-County Trial suggest that overdiagnosis is a minor phenomenon, more notable in patients of older age, and is primarily confined to the prevalent screen.[17] Prevalent screening may be more prone to detect indolent breast cancers, because cancers detected at incident screening indicate that the cancer is more biologically active and may be more likely to be clinically relevant. In fact, when Duffy and colleagues[21] evaluated the Two-County and Gothenburg RCT data, they found an estimated overdiagnosis rate of 1% for breast cancers diagnosed at incident screen after accounting for lead time. See **Table 1** for adjusted overdiagnosis estimates from randomized control trials.

Published RCT estimates of overdiagnosis are based on mammographic screening that was performed in an experimental setting at least 30 years ago. It would be informative to evaluate more recent clinical screening programs to investigate how time and technologic advances may have influenced overdiagnosis estimates from observational studies. de Gelder and colleagues[20] estimated overdiagnosis based on clinical data from 1990 to 2006 in the Netherlands, and found that the overdiagnosis risk ranged between 2.8% and 9.7%. Puliti and colleagues and the EURO-SCREEN Working Group analyzed 13 observational studies from 7 European countries that

Table 1
Overdiagnosis estimates from selected randomized control trials

Randomized Control Trial	Country	Patient Age at Randomization	Overdiagnosis (Invasive and DCIS)	Reference
Malmo	Sweden	55–69	10.5%	Zackrisson et al,[15] 2006
Swedish Two County	Sweden	40–69	RR 1.0	Yen et al, [17] 2012
CNBSS-1	Canada	40–49	12.4%	Marmot et al, [18] 2013
CNBSS-2	Canada	50–59	9.7%	Marmot et al, [18] 2013

estimated breast cancer overdiagnosis in clinical screening programs extending to 2006. Overdiagnosis estimates that adjusted for breast cancer risk and lead time ranged from 1% to 10%.[12] Unadjusted estimates, however, ranged from 0% to 54%. In general, overdiagnosis estimates that adjust for lead time are similar to those of the Malmö trial and EUROSCREEN Group. Studies that do not adjust for these factors tend to have higher estimates of overdiagnosis. Some of the other discrepancies seen between overdiagnosis estimates could be explained by differences in the patient denominators used, the length of follow up, and no lead time adjustment. For example, evaluating incidence data from several clinical screening programs in Europe, Canada, and Australia, Jorgensen and colleagues[13] estimated a much higher overdiagnosis rate of 52% (95% CI = 46%–58%). However, as Kopans points out, the expected cancer incidence may have been underestimated, because the background cancer incidence rates were considered stable[16] and adjustment was not made for rising background incidence. Furthermore, focusing on the screening uptake phase of the study can lead to a high observed incidence that cannot be accounted for by the lead time because of prevalence screening effect.[11] Evaluating the clinical screening program in Denmark, Jorgensen and colleagues[13] published an overdiagnosis estimate of 33%, but when Njor and colleagues[22] evaluated the same Danish screening program, they found a rate of only 2.3% (95% CI −3% to 8%) when the follow-up period was extended to account for lead time (**Table 2**).

Assumptions that Affect Overdiagnosis Estimates

Multiple factors affect overdiagnosis estimates, which has led to the wide range of the reported estimates. Factors that influence breast cancer overdiagnosis estimation include: temporal trends in background disease incidence, mammographic

lead time, follow-up period to account for lead time, age and cancer risk of the screened population, and whether ductal carcinoma in situ (DCIS) is included in the estimation. In a 2015 American Cancer Society publication, Oeffinger and colleagues[23] note that lower estimates of overdiagnosis risk are based on studies that "included adequate follow-up, had a control group or data on the incidence expected in the absence of screening, and properly adjusted for lead time as well as age."

Background incidence

An important variable that must be addressed when estimating breast cancer overdiagnosis is background incidence trend. The expected incidence of breast cancer absent screening is critical to a reliable overdiagnosis estimate. Increased breast cancer diagnoses as a result of increasing background incidence would declare themselves in both screened and unscreened women, and would not be due to screening. Over 40 years, the annual incidence of breast cancer in the United States prior to screening mammography was increasing 1.2% per year according to the Connecticut Tumor Registry.[4] Since that time, the background incidence may have increased further because of breast cancer risk factors such as environmental and dietary changes, increased obesity prevalence, and decreased/delayed parity.[24] Overdiagnosis estimates that assume a stable or low annual background incidence would be too high, since the expected incidence of breast cancer without screening would be too low. For example, in 2012, Bleyer and colleagues[25] evaluated Surveillance, Epidemiology, and End Results (SEER) breast cancer data over a 30-year period and published an estimated overdiagnosis rate of 31%. However, the authors utilized an annual background increase of 0.25% per year. A background incidence assumption of 0.25% for an unscreened patient population over 30 years would lead to a low expected incidence of breast cancer

Table 2
Overdiagnosis estimates from selected observational studies

Observational Study	Country	Patient Age at Randomization	Overdiagnosis (Invasive + DCIS)	Reference
Puliti	Italy	50–69	1-10%	Puliti et al, [12] 2012
Njor	Denmark	56–69	2.3%	Njor et al, [22] 2013
deGelder	Netherlands	50–69	2.8-9.7%	Puliti et al, [12] 2012; and de Gelder et al,[20] 2011

compared with the observed incidence, which would inflate the overdiagnosis estimate. Johnson and colleagues[26] subsequently reported that the incidence of advanced disease among women younger than 40 years of age has increased 2.07% per year. This is a population that is not routinely screened, yet experiencing increased background incidence of late stage breast cancer of greater than 2% per year. Environmental and biologic influences affecting breast cancer incidence in the unscreened patient population younger than 40 years of age are also likely contributing to an increased background incidence for women over the age of 40. Therefore, a background incidence rate of 0.25% increase per year for unscreened women older than 40 years of age is likely low. In 2014, Helvie and colleagues[14] examined long-term breast cancer incidence data from the prescreening era from SEER, Connecticut Tumor Registry, and United Kingdom data. The annual percentage change (APC) of breast cancer incidence ranged from 0.8% to 2.3%. Using a central estimate of 1.3% APC, the adjusted total breast cancer incidence increased by 7% over 30 years. However, as the authors point out, the increase should not be misconstrued as an overdiagnosis rate, because this incidence change would be further reduced when adjusted for lead time.

Lead time

Lead time is another factor that must be addressed when considering overdiagnosis. Lead time is the interval from screen detection of a breast cancer to when its clinical presentation would have been (absent screening). In general, lead times are shorter in premenopausal women than postmenopausal women. Mean lead times are approximately 1 to 2 years in premenopausal women and 3 to 4 years in postmenopausal women.[11] Mammographic lead times are thought to be exponentially distributed, meaning that most breast cancers have a relatively short lead time, but a decreasing proportion of breast cancers have an extended lead time.[11] de Gelder and colleagues[20] reported that approximately 20% of all tumors have a lead time of more than 5 years, and 5% will have a lead time of more than 10 years. To correctly adjust for this range of lead times, screened and nonscreened patients should be followed for years after the cessation of screening in order to properly render an overdiagnosis estimate. Because some patients have breast cancers with long lead times, it is essential to follow the patients long past the upper age limit of screening on the order of decades rather than years.[11] The importance of length of follow-up has been shown previously with data from the Malmö trial. Moss reported an overdiagnosis rate of 31% when the trial was ongoing.[27] However, Zackrisson and colleagues[15] found an overdiagnosis rate of 10% 15 years after the trial in women aged 55 to 69 years. Marmot and colleagues[18] followed 3 RCTs out for a period of 13 years, and among older women found an overdiagnosis rate of 10.7% for invasive and in situ disease. The time at which overdiagnosis is estimated can influence the estimate. Overdiagnosis estimates peaked during the implementation phase of screening,[18,20] owing to prevalence effect and a higher observed breast cancer incidence at that time. Patient age at screening also has a significant contribution to overdiagnosis estimations. Certainly, there is a subset of patients whose lead time is longer than their lifespan. According to a study done by Hendrick assuming variable patient ages and lead times, Type I overdiagnosis rates depend on a woman's age at the time of screening. For example, his overdiagnosis estimates ranged from less than 1% at age 40 (all lead times) to 22.5% at age 80 (mean lead time 40 months).[9] Hendrick's estimates confirm that Type I breast cancer overdiagnosis affects older women more, because their probability of dying from causes other than breast cancer is substantially higher than that of a 40- to 60-year-old woman.

Ductal carcinoma in situ

Because of the uncertainty regarding DCIS progression, it is advisable to consider whether DCIS has been included or separated from invasive carcinoma in an overdiagnosis estimate.[14] Following the introduction of screening mammography, DCIS now accounts for approximately 25% of breast cancers diagnosed. DCIS is a nonobligatory precursor to invasive breast cancer. Currently, there is no pathologic marker to predict which cases of DCIS will progress to invasive cancer. All grades of DCIS have the potential to progress to invasive disease, although low- and intermediate-grade DCIS may do so over a longer interval.[28] Because DCIS may have a longer mammographic lead time than invasive carcinoma, DCIS may be more likely to be characterized as overdiagnosis. Whether noninvasive disease is included in the calculation affects overdiagnosis estimates. For example, when examining data from the Gothenburg and Swedish Two-County Trials, Duffy and colleagues[21] reported that the upper limit overdiagnosis estimate for DCIS versus all cancers was 18% versus 2%, respectively (Gothenburg) and 16% versus 1% (Two-County), respectively. Although DCIS detection contributes to elevated overdiagnosis estimates, there are also data to support that the detection and treatment of DCIS prevents invasive cancer in some women. For example, Duffy and colleagues[21] reported that excess DCIS in the study arm was compensated for by a deficit in invasive disease[16] in the Gothenburg and Swedish Two-County trials. Furthermore, in the Two-County Trial, 12% of all deaths prevented were estimated to have resulted from the detection of DCIS.[29] More recently, Duffy and colleagues reported a significant negative association between the number of DCIS cases detected at screening and the number of invasive cancers that occurred in the subsequent 3-year interval. His group analyzed data from 5,243,658 women in the United Kingdom National Health Service Breast Screening Programme, and observed that up to a median DCIS detection rate of 1.5 cases per 1000 population, there was approximately 1 fewer invasive interval cancer case per 1.5 to 3 cases of DCIS.[30] These data suggest that the detection and treatment of DCIS prevent subsequent invasive breast cancer. Therefore, its detection is of benefit for some women.

FALSE-POSITIVE BIOPSY AND MAMMOGRAM

A false-positive biopsy (FPB) occurs when a recommendation for biopsy of a mammographic detected finding results in a benign pathologic result. Biopsy recommendation should always follow dedicated diagnostic imaging. The frequency of FPB has been estimated as 7.0% per decade when annual screening begins at age 40 and 9.4% per decade when screening begins at age 50.[31] On average, less than 1% per year of women who are getting screened annually get an FPB. Furthermore, the FPB rate has been shown to decrease as regular screening rounds increase. Blanchard and colleagues[32] showed the FPB rate decreased to 0.25% per year after 7 screening years, a value even less than unscreened women. Breast radiologists have markedly reduced the morbidity of breast biopsy over the last several decades. Biopsies are now nearly always performed with image-guided needle biopsy with local anesthesia, resulting in minimal scarring and post-biopsy recovery time. Although benign, some FPBs demonstrate high risk or premalignant conditions such as atypia, which allow for augmented surveillance or preventive therapeutics. When balancing life years gained versus risk of FPB by screening, Arleo and colleagues[33] determined that 1.0 life year is gained for every FPB.

When a woman is recalled from screening for additional imaging, the US Food and Drug Administration (FDA) refers to this as an "incomplete" mammogram. Additional imaging with diagnostic mammogram and/or ultrasound is indicated to complete the imaging evaluation. If a breast cancer is not diagnosed, the screening mammogram is often referred to as a false positive. A false positive is commonly referenced as a harm of screening because of the anxiety it may cause patients and utilization of limited health care resources. A false-positive screening mammogram over the course of a woman's screening arc is not uncommon. The chance of a false-positive result after 1 mammogram ranges from 7% to 12% in the United States,[34] and is higher for patients getting their baseline mammogram or screening sporadically. After 10 annual mammograms, the chance of having had 1 false-positive mammogram during that time is about 50% to 60%.[35] A false-positive result can cause anxiety for the patient that may persist, depending on the level of invasiveness of the subsequent workup.[35] However, the harm of a false-positive screening mammogram may be more of a concern to epidemiologists than patients. For example, when Schwartz and colleagues[36] surveyed 479 US women, they found that women are aware of the risks of false-positive results and view these risks as an acceptable consequence of screening. Sixty-three percent of the surveyed patients would tolerate 500 or more false positives for 1 life saved with screening, and 37% would tolerate

10,000 or more. It has been estimated that the actual number of false-positive mammograms for each life saved is between 30 and 200, assuming 2 to 6 lives saved for every 1000 women screened for 12 years.[37] Tosteson and colleagues[38] evaluated patients from the Digital Mammographic Imaging Screening Trial (DMIST) and found that false-positive mammograms were associated with increased short-term anxiety, but not long-term anxiety. Patients with a history of false-positive mammograms had a significantly increased future screening intention. However, it should be noted that the data from DMIST has the potential for selection bias. Continuing educational efforts for radiologists, patients, and referring clinicians may help to mitigate the level of distress associated with false-positive mammograms or biopsies.

RADIATION EXPOSURE

Both digital mammography (DM) and digital breast tomosynthesis (DBT) use low dose x-rays within FDA limits. A 2018 evaluation of mean glandular dose (MGD) from a single manufacturer's system found that the average MGD was 2.74 mGy for a 2-view study for each breast.[39] However, there is concern among some that radiation from serial mammography screening may cause breast cancer. Much of what is known about the risk of radiation-induced cancer is gleaned from studying high-dose cohorts in the years subsequent to their exposures. These studies have found a linear relationship between radiation dose and risk of radiation-induced cancers for estimated organ doses above 100 mGy. However, extrapolating the linear, no-threshold model to doses below 100 mGy is controversial.[40] Modeling performed by Miglioretti and colleagues[41] reported that annual screening of women aged 40 to 74 might induce a mean 125 breast cancer cases and 16 deaths, but avert 968 breast cancer deaths because of early detection. In this scenario, 8 breast cancer deaths would be averted per case of radiation-induced breast cancer. Yaffe and colleagues also modeled radiation-associated breast cancer risk assuming a 3.7 mGy dose to both breasts, 24% screening associated mortality reduction, and the ACS recommended screening schedule. He reported benefits in terms of breast cancer deaths averted because of screening (497 deaths per 100 000 women) and risks in terms of breast cancer deaths caused by radiation from screening (10.7 deaths per 100 000 women), which yielded a benefit-to-radiation-risk estimate of 47:1.[42] In 2020, Hendrick reported that the current 2-view MGD to an average breast from DM of 3 mGy has the same risk of causing cancer as approximately 6 weeks of natural background radiation.[40] Overall, the benefit-to-radiation-risk estimates are favorable for screening mammography. Nonetheless, radiologists, technologists, and physicists should work together to minimize patient dose whenever possible.

SUMMARY

In conclusion, screening mammography is an imperfect examination, but is currently the best tool available for the early detection of breast cancer when treatment options and survival are more favorable. The important mortality benefit offered by screening participation should not be eclipsed by its risks. Duffy and colleagues[43] reported a 30% mortality reduction with screening in the UK, and concluded that 2 to 2.5 lives were saved for every case that was estimated to have been overdiagnosed. At this time, the potential underdiagnosis of breast cancer without screening poses a more severe health risk to women than overdiagnosis. As understanding of breast cancer progression and tailored treatments continues to evolve, overtreatment of certain nonharmful breast cancers will decrease. Work should continue on methods to mitigate the risks of breast cancer screening to improve specificity and reduce radiation exposure.

CLINICS CARE POINTS

- Breast cancer continues to be a substantial risk to women's health worldwide. Routine screening mammography is currently the best tool available for the early detection of breast cancer.
- When making a decision to screen for breast cancer, women should be informed of the potential risks of screening in order to make a risk-benefit judgement that best suits their values.
- Overdiagnosis is a potential risk of breast cancer screening. It is more of a risk for older women due to competing mortality causes.
- Benefit to radiation-risk estimates are favorable in support of screening mammography.

DISCLOSURE

Dr M.A. Helvie has an institutional research grant from General Electric Healthcare for an activity not associated with this work. Dr C.H. Neal has no disclosures.

REFERENCES

1. Siegel RL, Miller KD, Jemal A. Cancer statistics, 2020. CA Cancer J Clin 2020;70:7–30.
2. Siegel RL, Miller KD, Jemal A. Cancer statistics, 2019. CA Cancer J Clin 2019;69:7–34.
3. Plevritis SK, Munoz D, Kurian AW, et al. Association of screening and treatment with breast cancer mortality by molecular subtype in US women, 2000-2012. JAMA 2018;319:154–64.
4. Helvie MA, Chang JT, Hendrick RE, et al. Reduction in late-stage breast cancer incidence in the mammography era: implications for overdiagnosis of invasive cancer. Cancer 2014;120:2649–56.
5. Hendrick RE, Baker JA, Helvie MA. Breast cancer deaths averted over 3 decades. Cancer 2019;125:1482–8.
6. Tabár L, Dean PB, Chen TH, et al. The incidence of fatal breast cancer measures the increased effectiveness of therapy in women participating in mammography screening. Cancer 2019;125:515–23.
7. Qaseem A, Lin JS, Mustafa RA, et al. Screening for breast cancer in average risk women: a guidance statement from the American College of Physicians. Ann Intern Med 2019;170:547–60.
8. Harding C, Pompei F, Burmistov D, et al. Breast cancer screening, incidence, and mortality across US counties. JAMA Intern Med 2015;175:1483–9.
9. Hendrick RE. Obligate overdiagnosis due to mammographic screening: a direct estimate for US women. Radiology 2018;287:391–7.
10. Arleo EA, Monticciolo DL, Monsees B, et al. Persistent untreated screening-detected breast cancer: an argument against delaying screening or increasing the interval between screenings. J Am Coll Radiol 2017;14:863–7.
11. Monticciolo DL, Helvie MA, Hendrick RE, et al. Current issues in the overdiagnosis and overtreatment of breast cancer. AJR Am J Roentgenol 2018;210:285–91.
12. Puliti D, Duffy SW, Miccinesi G, et al. Overdiagnosis in mammographic screening for breast cancer in Europe: a literature review. J Med Screen 2012;19(Suppl1):42–56.
13. Jørgensen KJ, Gøtzsche PC. Overdiagnosis in publicly organised mammography screening programmes: systematic review of incidence trends. BMJ 2009;339:b2587.
14. Helvie MA. Perspectives on the overdiagnosis of breast cancer associated with mammographic screening. J Breast Imaging 2019;1:278–82.
15. Zackrisson S, Andersson I, Janzon L, et al. Rate of over-diagnosis of breast cancer 15 years after end of Malmö mammographic screening trial: follow-up study. BMJ 2006;332:689–92.
16. Kopans DB, Smith RA, Duffy SW. Mammographic screening and "overdiagnosis." Radiology 2011;260:616–20.
17. Yen AM, Duffy SW, Chen TH, et al. Long-term incidence of breast cancer by trial arm in one county of the Swedish Two-County trial of mammographic screening. Cancer 2012;118:5728–32.
18. Marmot MG, Altman DG, Cameron DA, et al. The benefits and harms of breast cancer screening: an independent review. Br J Cancer 2013;108:2205–40.
19. Baines CJ, To T, Miller AB. Revised estimates of overdiagnosis from the Canadian national breast screening study. Prev Med 2016;90:66–71.
20. de Gelder R, Heijnsdijk EAM, van Ravesteyn NT, et al. Interpreting overdiagnosis estimates in population-based mammography screening. Epidemiol Rev 2011;33:111–21.
21. Duffy SW, Agbaje O, Tabar L, et al. Overdiagnosis and overtreatment of breast cancer: estimates of overdiagnosis from two trials of mammographic screening for breast cancer. Breast Cancer Res 2005;7:258–65.
22. Njor SH, Olsen AH, Blichert-Toft M, et al. Overdiagnosis in screening mammography in Denmark: population based cohort study. BMJ 2013;346:f1064.
23. Oeffinger KC, Fontham ETH, Etzioni R, et al. Breast cancer screening for women at average risk: 2015 guideline update from the American Cancer Society. JAMA 2015;314:1599–614.
24. Rojas K, Stuckey A. Breast cancer epidemiology and risk factors. Clin Obstet Gynecol 2016;59:651–72.
25. Bleyer A, Welch HG. Effect of three decades of screening mammography on breast-cancer incidence. N Engl J Med 2012;3 67:1998–2005.
26. Johnson RH, Chien FL, Bleyer A. Incidence of breast cancer with distant involvement among women in the United States, 1976 to 2009. JAMA 2013;309:800–5.
27. Moss S. Overdiagnosis in randomized controlled trials of breast cancer screening. Breast Cancer Res 2005;7:230–4.
28. Collins LC, Tamimi RM, Baer HJ, et al. Outcome of patients with ductal carcinoma in situ untreated after diagnostic biopsy: results from the Nurses' Health Study. Cancer 2005;103:1778–84.
29. Duffy SW, Tabar L, Vitak B, et al. The Relative contributions of screen-detected in situ and invasive breast carcinomas in reducing mortality from the disease. Eur J Cancer 2003;39:1755–60.
30. Duffy SW, Dibden A, Michalopoulos D, et al. Screen detection of ductal carcinoma in situ and subsequent incidence of invasive interval breast cancers: a retrospective population-based study. Lancet Oncol 2016;17(2):e46.

31. Siu AL. Screening for breast cancer: U.S. preventive services task force recommendation statement. Ann Intern Med 2016;164:279–96.

32. Blanchard K, Colbert JA, Kopans DB, et al. Long-term risk of false-positive screening results and subsequent biopsy as a function of mammography use. Radiology 2006;240:335–42.

33. Arleo EK, Hendrick RE, Helvie MA, et al. Comparison of recommendations for screening mammography using CISNET models. Cancer 2017;123:3673–80.

34. Nelson HD, Fu R, Cantor A, et al. Effectiveness of breast cancer screening: systematic review and meta-analysis to update the 2009 U.S. Preventive services task force recommendation. Ann Intern Med 2016;164:244–55.

35. Hubbard RA, Kerlikowske K, Flowers CI, et al. Cumulative probability of false-positive recall or biopsy recommendation after 10 years of screening mammography: a cohort study. Ann Intern Med 2011;155:481–92.

36. Schwartz LM, Woloshin S, Sox HC, et al. US women's attitudes to false-positive mammography results and detection of ductal carcinoma in situ: cross-sectional survey. BMJ 2000;320:1635–40.

37. Nyström 1 L, Rutqvist LE, Wall S, et al. Breast cancer screening with mammography: overview of Swedish randomised trials. Lancet 1993;341:973–8.

38. Tosteson ANA, Fryback DG, Hammond CS, et al. Consequences of false-positive screening mammograms. JAMA Intern Med 2014;174:954–61.

39. Gennaro G, Bernardi D, Houssami N. Radiation dose with digital breast tomosynthesis compared to digital mammography: per-view analysis. Eur Radiol 2018;28:573–81.

40. Hendrick RE. Radiation doses and risks in breast screening. J Breast Imaging 2020;1–13. https://doi.org/10.1093/jbi/wbaa016.

41. Miglioretti DL, Lange J, van den Broek JJ, et al. Radiation-induced breast cancer incidence and mortality from digital mammography screening. a modeling study. Ann Intern Med 2016;164:205–14.

42. Yaffe MJ, Mainprize JG. Risk of radiation-induced breast cancer from mammographic screening. Radiology 2011;258:98–105.

43. Duffy SW, Tabar L, Olsen A, et al. Absolute numbers of lives saved and overdiagnosis in breast cancer screening, from a randomized trial and from the breast screening programme in England. J Med Screen 2010;17:25–30.

Management of High-Risk Breast Lesions

Manisha Bahl, MD, MPH

KEYWORDS

- Atypical ductal hyperplasia • Atypical lobular hyperplasia • Breast cancer • Flat epithelial atypia
- High-risk lesion • Lobular carcinoma in situ • Papilloma • Radial scar

KEY POINTS

- High-risk breast lesions are a group of heterogeneous lesions that can be associated with a synchronous or adjacent breast cancer and that confer an increased lifetime risk of breast cancer.
- Surgical excision is typically recommended for atypical ductal hyperplasia (ADH), but small-volume ADH that is completely removed at core biopsy may be surveilled rather than excised in certain scenarios.
- Observation after risk assessment and multidisciplinary input may be appropriate for pure flat epithelial atypia, lobular neoplasia with imaging-pathologic concordance and adequate sampling, papillomas without atypia, and small radial scars.
- For women with a history of ADH or lobular hyperplasia and greater than 20% lifetime risk, clinical breast examination with risk-reduction counseling every 6 to 12 months and annual screening mammogram are recommended, in addition to consideration of annual breast MR imaging and chemoprevention.

INTRODUCTION

More than 10% of breast biopsies performed based on findings at mammography yield high-risk lesions (HRLs).[1] HRLs refer to a group of heterogeneous lesions that can be associated with a synchronous or adjacent breast cancer and that confer an elevated lifetime risk of breast cancer.[2,3] These lesions include atypical ductal hyperplasia (ADH), flat epithelial atypia (FEA), lobular hyperplasia (which refers to atypical lobular hyperplasia [ALH] and lobular carcinoma in situ [LCIS]), papillomas, and radial scars.

There are no universally agreed-on recommendations for the management of HRLs, which is thought to be due to variations in reported upgrade rates, limitations in study designs of available literature (eg, single-institution retrospective studies and selection bias with regard to which patients undergo surgical excision), lack of radiology-pathology concordance, and lack of consensus among pathologists regarding the diagnostic criteria for HRLs.[4,5] This lack of consensus has led to variations in patient care, with management after core needle biopsy including close imaging and clinical follow-up or excisional biopsy to evaluate for ductal carcinoma in situ (DCIS) and invasive cancer.[4–7] This article reviews histologic features and clinical presentation of each of the HRLs, current evidence with regard to management, and guidelines from the American Society of Breast Surgeons (ASBrS) and National Comprehensive Cancer Network (NCCN). In addition, imaging surveillance and risk-reduction strategies for women with HRLs are discussed.

HIGH-RISK LESIONS
Atypical Ductal Hyperplasia

ADH is characterized by the intraductal proliferation of uniform epithelial cells with monomorphic round nuclei that fill part of the involved duct or completely fill the duct but measure less than

Department of Radiology, Massachusetts General Hospital/Harvard Medical School, 55 Fruit Street, WAC 240, Boston, MA 02114, USA
E-mail address: mbahl1@mgh.harvard.edu

Radiol Clin N Am 59 (2021) 29–40
https://doi.org/10.1016/j.rcl.2020.08.005
0033-8389/21/© 2020 Elsevier Inc. All rights reserved.

radiologic.theclinics.com

2 mm or involve fewer than 2 ducts (**Fig. 1**).[8] ADH resembles low-grade DCIS with cytologic and architectural atypia but is of limited extent.[8] ADH typically presents in asymptomatic women as calcifications at mammography and less commonly as a mass at sonography (**Fig. 2**).[9] It can also be seen as non-mass enhancement at MR imaging.[10]

A meta-analysis of 93 studies found that the pooled upgrade rate of ADH to DCIS or invasive cancer was 29% (95% confidence interval, 26%–32%) for lesions that were surgically excised and 5% (95% confidence interval, 4%–8%) for lesions that were surveilled.[11] The invasive cancer upgrade rate was 9% (95% confidence interval, 7%–11%) for lesions that were surgically excised and 3.4% (95% confidence interval, 1.8%–6.4%) for lesions that were surveilled.[11] Risk factors associated with upgrade risk include age at biopsy, breast cancer risk, lesion size, presence of multiple lesions, needle gauge, and number of biopsies.[12]

Given the relatively high upgrade rate of ADH to cancer, and the challenge at pathology of distinguishing ADH from DCIS, the ASBrS and NCCN recommend surgical excision for most ADH.[13,14] However, per the ASBrS guidelines, small-volume ADH that is completely removed at core biopsy may be observed if the imaging findings and pathology results are concordant and after consideration of breast cancer risk factors and input of the multidisciplinary team.[13] Several models to predict upgrade risk of ADH have been developed, which can inform the decision-making process.[12,15–18] One institution proposed the following guidelines for surveillance rather than surgical excision of ADH: lesion smaller than 6 mm with complete removal of calcifications, smaller than 6 mm with incomplete removal of calcifications but 2 or fewer foci of ADH, or 6 to 21 mm with 2 or fewer foci of ADH.[19,20] Of 41 excised cases that met criteria for surveillance, only 1 was upgraded at surgery, for an upgrade rate of 2%.[20]

Flat Epithelial Atypia

FEA is characterized by the intraductal proliferation of epithelial cells with low-grade cytologic atypia, which demonstrate a "flat" pattern of growth along the ductal or acinar wall with no architecturally atypical structures.[21] The involved terminal duct-lobular units (TDLUs) are enlarged and dilated (**Fig. 3**).[21] ADH and DCIS demonstrate both cytologic and architectural atypia, whereas FEA is characterized by the presence of cytologic atypia without architectural atypia.[21] FEA typically presents in asymptomatic women as calcifications

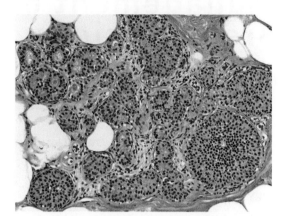

Fig. 1. Histologic features of ADH (hematoxylin-eosin, original magnification ×200), which is characterized by the intraductal proliferation of uniform epithelial cells with monomorphic round nuclei that fill part of the involved duct or completely fill the duct but measure less than 2 mm or involve fewer than 2 ducts. (*Courtesy of* Melinda Lerwill, MD, Department of Pathology, Massachusetts General Hospital, Boston, MA.)

at mammography, often grouped in distribution and amorphous in morphology (**Fig. 4**).[22] Less commonly, FEA can present as an irregular mass at sonography.[22]

In a meta-analysis of 32 studies, the upgrade rate of FEA to cancer at surgery was widely variable, ranging from 0% to 42%; the overall pooled upgrade rate estimate was 11.1%.[23] Among studies of higher quality, the overall pooled upgrade rate estimate was 7.5% (95% confidence interval, 5.4%–10.4%), and the invasive cancer upgrade rate was only 3% (95% confidence interval, 1.9%–4.5%).[23] Risk factors associated with an

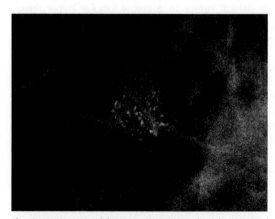

Fig. 2. A 45-year-old woman presented with grouped pleomorphic calcifications at mammography. Stereotactic core needle biopsy revealed ADH, which was upgraded to grade 1 DCIS at surgical excision.

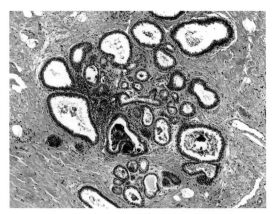

Fig. 3. Histologic features of FEA (hematoxylin-eosin, original magnification ×100), demonstrating variably dilated terminal duct-lobular units with secretions and calcifications lined by atypical cells. (*Courtesy of* Melinda Lerwill, MD, Department of Pathology, Massachusetts General Hospital, Boston, MA.)

increased cancer upgrade risk include a genetic mutation, the presence of concurrent ADH, ALH, or radial scar, and incomplete removal of the imaging finding at core needle biopsy.[24–27] In the aforementioned meta-analysis, the upgrade rate of FEA to ADH at surgery was also widely variable, ranging from 0% to 60%; the pooled upgrade rate estimate was 17.9% overall and 18.6% among studies of higher quality.[23]

Given the overall low cancer upgrade rate of FEA, and that upgraded cases are more often DCIS than invasive cancer, the ASBrS recommends observation with imaging and clinical follow-up of pure FEA.[13] Surgical excision is recommended for FEA with concurrent ADH.[13] Guidelines from the NCCN also indicate that pure

FEA may not require surgical excision, but specific criteria for surveillance versus surgical excision are not provided.[14] Although the ASBrS and NCCN favor surveillance of pure FEA, surgical excision may be warranted to evaluate for a higher-risk lesion (eg, ADH) to inform decision-making with regard to chemoprevention.[26]

Lobular Hyperplasia

The term lobular hyperplasia refers to ALH and LCIS. ALH and LCIS are characterized by the proliferation of dyshesive monomorphic epithelial cells, often with intracytoplasmic vacuoles, that arise within the TDLUs and distend the acini.[28] ALH is less extensive than LCIS, with ALH defined as involving less than 50% of the acini in a TDLU (**Figs. 5** and **6**).[28,29] Pleomorphic LCIS and florid LCIS are morphologic variants of LCIS: pleomorphic LCIS has high-grade cytologic features, and florid refers to an architectural growth pattern causing expansion of ducts and lobules.[30] ALH and LCIS are thought to represent incidental findings at core needle biopsy that are typically associated with calcifications (**Fig. 7**).[30–32] ADH and LCIS can also be seen as non-mass enhancement or as an enhancing mass at MR imaging.[33]

Several published studies report low overall upgrade rates of ALH and classic LCIS. For example, of 85 consecutive cases in which core needle biopsy yielded pure lobular neoplasia, upgrade rates to cancer were 3% (95% confidence interval, 0%–9%) for radiologic-pathologic concordant cases and 38% (95% confidence interval, 9%–76%) for

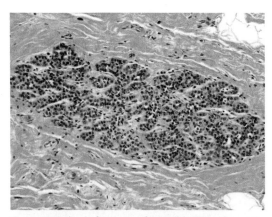

Fig. 5. Histologic features of ALH (hematoxylin-eosin, original magnification ×200), characterized by the proliferation of dyshesive monomorphic epithelial cells, often with intracytoplasmic vacuoles, that arise within the terminal duct-lobular units and distend the acini. ALH is less extensive than classic LCIS. (*Courtesy of* Melinda Lerwill, MD, Department of Pathology, Massachusetts General Hospital, Boston, MA.)

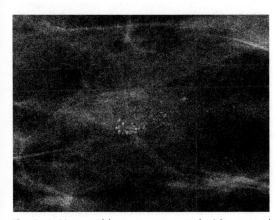

Fig. 4. A 41-year-old woman presented with grouped amorphous calcifications at screening mammography. Stereotactic core needle biopsy and surgical excision yielded FEA.

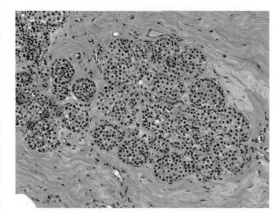

Fig. 6. Histologic features of classic LCIS (hematoxylin-eosin, original magnification ×200), characterized by the proliferation of dyshesive monomorphic epithelial cells, often with intracytoplasmic vacuoles, that arise within the terminal duct-lobular units and distend the acini. Classic LCIS is more extensive than ALH. (*Courtesy of* Melinda Lerwill, MD, Department of Pathology, Massachusetts General Hospital, Boston, MA.)

discordant cases.[34] Among 77 patients with pure lobular neoplasia, the upgrade rate to cancer was only 1% when reviewed by central pathology.[35] Among 68 patients with pure lobular neoplasia, no upgrades at surgery were observed in normal-risk patients with calcifications identified at mammographic screening.[36] Features associated with increased upgrade risk include radiologic-pathologic discordance, extensive LCIS with more than 4 foci, and imaging for high-risk indications.[34,36]

According to guidelines from the ASBrS, observation of ALH and LCIS can be offered in the setting of small-volume lesions, radiologic-pathologic concordance, and the absence of other HRLs.[13] Per guidelines from the NCCN, options for management of ALH and LCIS with radiologic-pathologic concordance include observation with imaging and clinical follow-up or surgical excision.[14] The increased risk of upgrade associated with multifocal/extensive LCIS involving more than 4 TDLUs is noted in the NCCN guidelines.[14] Surgical excision of higher-risk LCIS variants (ie, pleomorphic and florid LCIS) is widely recommended (**Fig. 8**).[13,14,29]

Papilloma

Intraductal papillomas are characterized by fibro-vascular cores lined by 2 cell types, an inner myoepithelial layer and an outer epithelial layer (**Fig. 9**).[37] Central papillomas, which are the most common type of papilloma, originate in the large ducts and are usually solitary, whereas peripheral papillomas arise in the TDLUs and can be multiple.[6] Papillomas can present with nipple discharge or as a palpable mass or can be discovered incidentally at imaging.[38] On imaging, papillomas manifest as a mass or calcifications at mammography, an intraluminal filling detect or duct dilatation at galactography, an intraductal mass at sonography, or an enhancing mass at MR imaging (**Fig. 10**).[37]

In a meta-analysis of 34 studies, which included more than 2000 nonmalignant papillary lesions, the pooled upgrade rate to cancer was 15.7% (95% confidence interval, 12.8%–18.5%).[39] The upgrade rate of papillomas with atypia was

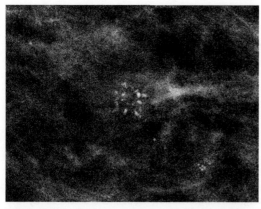

Fig. 7. A 76-year-old woman presented with grouped pleomorphic calcifications at screening mammography. Stereotactic core needle biopsy yielded fibroadenomatous stromal change with associated stromal microcalcifications with a focus of incidental ALH. Surgical excision yielded only focal ALH.

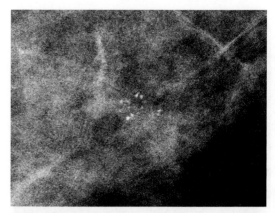

Fig. 8. A 42-year-old woman presented with grouped amorphous calcifications at screening mammography. Stereotactic core needle biopsy revealed pleomorphic LCIS, which was upgraded to grade 2 invasive lobular carcinoma at surgical excision.

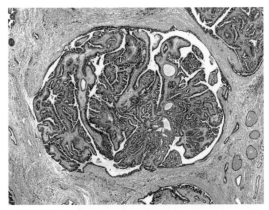

Fig. 9. Histologic features of papilloma (hematoxylin-eosin, original magnification ×50), demonstrating a well-developed fibrovascular core. (*Courtesy of* Melinda Lerwill, MD, Department of Pathology, Massachusetts General Hospital, Boston, MA.)

36.9% (95% confidence interval, 29.5%–44.3%), whereas the upgrade rate of papillomas without atypia was only 7.0% (95% confidence interval, 5.6%–8.3%).[39] Another review reported similar upgrade rates of 34% for papillomas with atypia and 7.6% without atypia.[40] In a recent study of 500 women with papillary lesions, the upgrade rate to cancer was reported to be 1.8% (95% confidence interval, 0.9%–3.4%).[41] Apart from atypia, features associated with increased upgrade risk include peripheral location, large size, bloody nipple discharge, and palpability.[42,43]

Given the high upgrade rate, surgical excision is widely recommended for papillomas with atypia.[13,39,40] Per the ASBrS, the decision to excise versus observe a papilloma without atypia should be based on assessment of the individual's risk level, including such criteria as breast cancer risk factors, lesion size, presence of nipple discharge, and palpability, although palpability alone is not considered to be an absolute indication for surgical excision.[13] Incidental, benign papillomas can be observed with close imaging and clinical follow-up.[13] Guidelines from the NCCN also indicate that papillomas without atypia may not require surgical excision, but specific criteria for surveillance versus surgical excision are not provided.[14]

Radial Scar

Radial scars are characterized by a central focus of fibroelastotic stroma with epithelial elements entrapped within the stroma.[44] The distortion of entrapped glands combined with the stellate appearance of radial scars can mimic cancers at imaging and pathologic examination (**Fig. 11**).[44]

Of note, radial scar typically refers to lesions smaller than 1 cm, whereas complex sclerosing lesion typically refers to lesions larger than 1 cm, although these terms can also be used interchangeably.[45,46] Historically, radial scars have been referred to as radial sclerosing lesions, sclerosing papillary proliferations, nonencapsulated sclerosing lesions, and indurative mastopathy.[47] Radial scars typically present as architectural distortion at mammography, which is more frequently detected at digital breast tomosynthesis when compared with 2-dimensional digital mammography (**Fig. 12**).[48] Radial scars can also present as calcifications at mammography.[45] When seen at ultrasound, radial scars most often appear as irregular hypoechoic masses.[45]

According to a meta-analysis of 49 studies that included more than 3000 radial scars with surgical outcomes, the random-effects pooled estimate of upgrade rate to cancer was 7% (95% confidence interval, 5%–9%).[49] Of the upgraded cases, 66% upgraded to DCIS.[49] Radial scars without atypia and assessed by 8-gauge to 11-gauge vacuum-assisted biopsies had an upgrade rate of only 1% (95% confidence interval, 0%–4%) to DCIS.[49] Features associated with increased upgrade risk include older age, postmenopausal status, the finding of architectural distortion or mass (rather than calcifications), the presence of atypia, and small biopsy gauge.[49–51] Despite the increased identification of radial scars manifesting as architectural distortion with tomosynthesis, no differences in upgrade rates to cancer have been observed before and after the introduction of tomosynthesis.[52,53]

Given the relatively low upgrade rate of radial scar to cancer, observation with imaging and clinical follow-up is considered to be reasonable for adequately sampled radial scars with radiologic-pathologic concordance.[13,14,46] In particular, follow-up is appropriate for small, imaging-detected or incidental radial scars with multidisciplinary input; however, it may be challenging to assess changes in radial scars presenting as architectural distortion, and thus very close attention at follow-up is advised if surveillance rather than surgical excision is pursued.[13] MR imaging has also been used for problem-solving purposes for radial scars identified at mammography and could help triage which biopsy-proven radial scars require excision and which can be safely observed; however, radial scars may enhance at MR imaging even without associated cancer.[45] Similar to FEA, surgical excision may be warranted to assess for a higher-risk lesion, with reported upgrade rates to a higher-risk lesion exceeding 20%, to guide patient discussion regarding chemoprevention.[51,53]

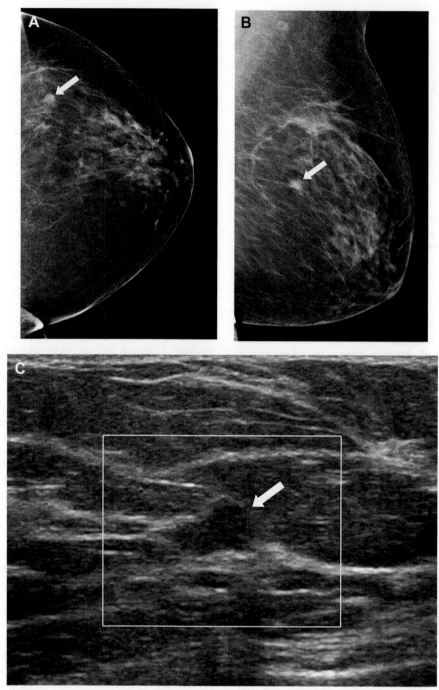

Fig. 10. A 65-year-old woman presented with a mass at screening mammography. (*A*) Left craniocaudal view and (*B*) left mediolateral oblique view demonstrate a mass in the upper outer quadrant of the breast at posterior depth (*arrows*). (*C*) Ultrasound demonstrates an irregular hypoechoic mass (*arrow*), which corresponds to the mammographic mass. Ultrasound-guided core needle biopsy yielded a papilloma with atypia, which was upgraded to a papilloma with grade 2 DCIS.

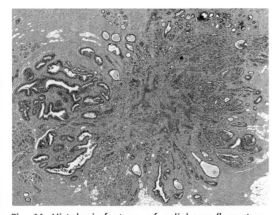

Fig. 11. Histologic features of radial scar (hematoxylin-eosin, original magnification ×50), which has a stellate appearance and is characterized by a central focus of fibroelastotic stroma with epithelial elements entrapped within the stroma. (*Courtesy of* Melinda Lerwill, MD, Department of Pathology, Massachusetts General Hospital, Boston, MA.)

Summary of Management Guidelines

Table 1 summarizes guidelines for the management of HRLs from the ASBrS.[13] A multidisciplinary approach for HRL management recommendations is advocated. For example, at The University of Texas M.D. Anderson Cancer Center in Houston, Texas, a multidisciplinary conference is held every week with breast cancer specialists (radiologists, surgeons, and pathologists) to discuss each patient with an HRL diagnosis and to issue personalized recommendations.[38,54,55] The following variables are taken into consideration: clinical variables (eg, age and risk factors for breast cancer), imaging variables (eg, lesion size and adequacy of sampling), and pathologic variables (eg, concordance of pathologic and imaging findings and lesion extent).[38] For example, focal ADH with near complete removal of the calcifications at core biopsy may lead to a recommendation for imaging surveillance

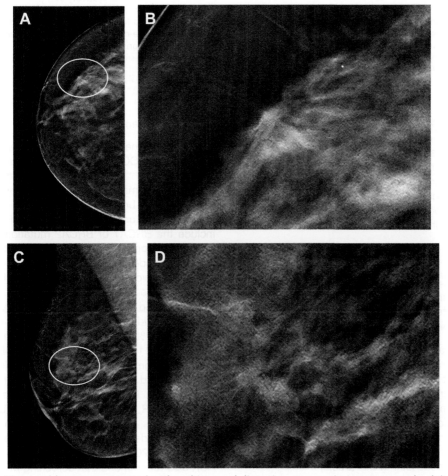

Fig. 12. A 50-year-old woman presented with architectural distortion at screening mammography. (*A*) Right craniocaudal tomosynthesis view, (*B*) magnified right craniocaudal tomosynthesis view, (*C*) right mediolateral oblique tomosynthesis view, and (*D*) magnified right mediolateral oblique tomosynthesis view demonstrate architectural distortion in the upper outer quadrant at middle depth (*circles*). Stereotactic core needle biopsy yielded a radial scar. Surgical excision was not performed.

Table 1
Consensus guidelines on the management of high-risk lesions (HRLs) from the American Society of Breast Surgeons

HRL	Recommendation	Exceptions/Notes
Atypical ductal hyperplasia (ADH)	Surgical excision	Surveillance okay if ADH is small-volume and completely removed at core needle biopsy and based on risk factor assessment and multidisciplinary input
Flat epithelial atypia (FEA)	Surveillance	Surgical excision if concurrent ADH
Lobular neoplasia (atypical lobular hyperplasia [ALH] or lobular carcinoma in situ [LCIS][a])	Surgical excision or surveillance	Surgical excision if there is radiology-pathology discordance, limited sampling, or other HRL is present
Papillary lesion	Surgical excision or surveillance	Surgical excision if palpable or if associated atypia, surveillance okay if incidental and no associated atypia
Radial scar	Surgical excision	Surveillance okay if small and adequately sampled

[a] This recommendation applies to classic LCIS. Surgical excision is recommended for pleomorphic and florid LCIS.
Adapted from the American Society of Breast Surgeons. Consensus guideline on concordance assessment of image-guided breast biopsies and management of borderline or high-risk lesions, 2016. Available at: https://www.breastsurgeons.org/docs/statements/Consensus-Guideline-on-Concordance-Assessment-of-Image-Guided-Breast-Biopsies.pdf. Accessed May 1, 2020; with permission.

rather than surgical excision, in addition to consultation for breast cancer risk-reduction options.[38] Prior studies have evaluated the diagnostic utility of MR imaging to exclude the presence of coexisting cancer in the setting of an HRL.[56–58] Machine learning models that combine patient, imaging, and pathology data to predict risk of HRL upgrade are also being explored.[12,59]

BREAST CANCER RISK REDUCTION
Active Surveillance

For women with a history of ADH, ALH, or LCIS and greater than 20% lifetime risk, guidelines from the NCCN recommend the following[14]:

- Clinical breast examination, risk assessment, and risk-reduction counseling every 6 to 12 months
- Screening mammogram (with consideration of tomosynthesis) every year
- Consideration of breast MR imaging every year (discussed in the following section)
- Consideration of risk-reduction strategies (discussed later in this article)[60]
- Patient familiarity with her own breasts (ie, breast awareness)

Breast MR imaging

Current guidelines by the American Cancer Society (ACS),[61] NCCN,[14] and the American College of Radiology (ACR)[62] recommend annual screening MR imaging for women with an elevated lifetime risk of breast cancer, primarily based on hereditary factors. Indications for MR imaging include the *BRCA1* or *BRCA2* mutation and lifetime risk of approximately 20% to 25% or greater based on models that are largely based on family history. For women with ADH, ALH, or LCIS, the ACS concluded that there is not enough evidence to recommend for or against screening MR imaging.[61] The guidelines note a lifetime risk of breast cancer of 10% to 20% in women with LCIS or ALH, a 6-fold to 10-fold increased risk of invasive cancer in women with LCIS, and a 4-fold to 5-fold increased risk of invasive cancer in women with ADH.[61] Per guidelines from the NCCN, screening MR imaging should be considered for women with ADH, ALH, or LCIS based on emerging evidence, if lifetime risk is greater than or equal to 20%.[14] Recent guidelines from the ACR also recommend that screening MR imaging be considered for women with ADH, ALH, or LCIS, especially if other risk factors are present.[62]

Risk-Reduction Strategies

For women with a history of ADH, ALH, or LCIS and life expectancy of 10 or more years, guidelines from the NCCN recommend risk-reducing counseling.[60] Lifestyle modifications, such as limiting alcohol consumption, exercising, and maintaining a healthy weight, are encouraged.[60] If risk-reducing therapy is desired, then tamoxifen is recommended for premenopausal women, and tamoxifen, raloxifene, anastrozole, or exemestane is recommended for postmenopausal women.[60] The benefits of risk-reducing therapy in women with FEA are not supported by robust data, but consideration can be given to these agents if 5-year breast cancer risk is 1.7% or higher and if life expectancy is 10 years or more.[60]

SUMMARY

HRLs refer to a group of heterogeneous lesions that can be associated with a synchronous or adjacent breast cancer and that confer an elevated lifetime risk of breast cancer. The lack of consensus regarding management of HRLs had led to variations in patient care, with options after core needle biopsy including close imaging and clinical follow-up or excisional biopsy to evaluate for cancer. For ADH, surgical excision is generally recommended, but small-volume ADH that is completely excised at core biopsy may be observed if the imaging findings and pathology results are concordant and after breast cancer risk assessment and multidisciplinary input. Clinical and imaging follow-up after breast cancer risk assessment and multidisciplinary input may be appropriate for other HRLs, including pure FEA, lobular neoplasia (ALH and LCIS) wlth imaging-pathologic concordance and adequate sampling, nonpalpable papillomas without atypia, and small radial scars with adequate sampling. For women with a history of ADH, ALH, or LCIS and greater than 20% lifetime risk, clinical breast examination with risk-reduction counseling every 6 to 12 months and annual screening mammogram are recommended, in addition to consideration of annual breast MR imaging and risk-reduction strategies, including chemoprevention.

CLINICS CARE POINTS

- HRLs refer to a group of heterogeneous lesions that can be associated with a synchronous or adjacent breast cancer and that confer an elevated lifetime risk of breast cancer.

- Surgical excision is typically recommended for ADH, but small-volume ADH completely removed at core biopsy may be observed if the imaging findings and pathology results are concordant and based on breast cancer risk factor assessment and multidisciplinary input.
- Imaging and clinical follow-up after breast cancer risk assessment and multidisciplinary input may be appropriate for the following:
  ○ FEA without concurrent ADH
  ○ Lobular neoplasia (ALH and classic LCIS) with imaging-pathologic concordance, adequate sampling, and the absence of a concurrent high-risk lesion
  ○ Nonpalpable papillomas without atypia
  ○ Small, adequately sampled radial scars
- For women with a history of ADH or lobular neoplasia and greater than 20% lifetime risk, clinical breast examination with risk-reduction counseling every 6 to 12 months and annual screening mammogram are recommended, in addition to consideration of annual breast MR imaging and risk-reduction strategies (including chemoprevention).

DISCLOSURE

The author has no disclosures.

REFERENCES

1. Eby PR, Ochsner JE, DeMartini WB, et al. Is surgical excision necessary for focal atypical ductal hyperplasia found at stereotactic vacuum-assisted breast biopsy? Ann Surg Oncol 2008;15(11):3232–8.
2. Degnim AC, King TA. Surgical management of high-risk breast lesions. Surg Clin North Am 2013;93(2): 329–40.
3. Boateng S, Tirada N, Khorjekar G, et al. Excision or observation: the dilemma of managing high-risk breast lesions. Curr Probl Diagn Radiol 2020;49(2): 124–32.
4. Georgian-Smith D, Lawton TJ. Variations in physician recommendations for surgery after diagnosis of a high-risk lesion on breast core needle biopsy. AJR Am J Roentgenol 2012;198(2):256–63.
5. Falomo E, Adejumo C, Carson KA, et al. Variability in the management recommendations given for high-risk breast lesions detected on image-guided core needle biopsy at U.S. academic institutions. Curr Probl Diagn Radiol 2019;48(5):462–6.
6. Gulla S, Lancaster R, De Los Santos J. High-risk breast lesions and current management. Semin Roentgenol 2018;53(4):252–60.
7. Kappel C, Seely J, Watters J, et al. A survey of Canadian breast health professionals' recommendations

for high-risk benign breast disease. Can J Surg 2019;
62(5):358–60.

8. Kader T, Hill P, Rakha EA, et al. Atypical ductal hyperplasia: update on diagnosis, management, and molecular landscape. Breast Cancer Res 2018; 20(1):39.

9. Mesurolle B, Perez JC, Azzumea F, et al. Atypical ductal hyperplasia diagnosed at sonographically guided core needle biopsy: frequency, final surgical outcome, and factors associated with underestimation. AJR Am J Roentgenol 2014;202(6):1389–94.

10. Tsuchiya K, Mori N, Schacht DV, et al. Value of breast MRI for patients with a biopsy showing atypical ductal hyperplasia (ADH). J Magn Reson Imaging 2017;46(6):1738–47.

11. Schiaffino S, Calabrese M, Melani EF, et al. Upgrade rate of percutaneously diagnosed pure atypical ductal hyperplasia: systematic review and meta-analysis of 6458 lesions. Radiology 2020;294(1): 76–86.

12. Harrington L, diFlorio-Alexander R, Trinh K, et al. Prediction of atypical ductal hyperplasia upgrades through a machine learning approach to reduce unnecessary surgical excisions. JCO Clin Cancer Inform 2018;2:1–11.

13. The American Society of Breast Surgeons. Consensus guideline on concordance assessment of image-guided breast biopsies and management of borderline or high-risk lesions. 2016. Available at: https://www.breastsurgeons.org/docs/statements/Consensus-Guideline-on-Concordance-Assessment-of-Image-Guided-Breast-Biopsies.pdf. Accessed May 1, 2020.

14. NCCN Clinical Practice Guidelines in Oncology. Breast cancer screening and diagnosis, version 1.2019. Available at: https://www.nccn.org/professionals/physician_gls/pdf/breast-screening.pdf. Accessed May 1, 2020.

15. Ko E, Han W, Lee JW, et al. Scoring system for predicting malignancy in patients diagnosed with atypical ductal hyperplasia at ultrasound-guided core needle biopsy. Breast Cancer Res Treat 2008; 112(1):189–95.

16. Nguyen CV, Albarracin CT, Whitman GJ, et al. Atypical ductal hyperplasia in directional vacuum-assisted biopsy of breast microcalcifications: considerations for surgical excision. Ann Surg Oncol 2011;18(3):752–61.

17. Khoury T, Li Z, Sanati S, et al. The risk of upgrade for atypical ductal hyperplasia detected on magnetic resonance imaging-guided biopsy: a study of 100 cases from four academic institutions. Histopathology 2016;68(5):713–21.

18. Pena A, Shah SS, Fazzio RT, et al. Multivariate model to identify women at low risk of cancer upgrade after a core needle biopsy diagnosis of atypical ductal hyperplasia. Breast Cancer Res Treat 2017;164(2): 295–304.

19. Forgeard C, Benchaib M, Guerin N, et al. Is surgical biopsy mandatory in case of atypical ductal hyperplasia on 11-gauge core needle biopsy? A retrospective study of 300 patients. Am J Surg 2008; 196(3):339–45.

20. Caplain A, Drouet Y, Peyron M, et al. Management of patients diagnosed with atypical ductal hyperplasia by vacuum-assisted core biopsy: a prospective assessment of the guidelines used at our institution. Am J Surg 2014;208(2):260–7.

21. Lerwill MF. Flat epithelial atypia of the breast. Arch Pathol Lab Med 2008;132(4):615–21.

22. Solorzano S, Mesurolle B, Omeroglu A, et al. Flat epithelial atypia of the breast: pathological-radiological correlation. AJR Am J Roentgenol 2011;197(3):740–6.

23. Rudin AV, Hoskin TL, Fahy A, et al. Flat epithelial atypia on core biopsy and upgrade to cancer: a systematic review and meta-analysis. Ann Surg Oncol 2017;24(12):3549–58.

24. Peres A, Barranger E, Becette V, et al. Rates of upgrade to malignancy for 271 cases of flat epithelial atypia (FEA) diagnosed by breast core biopsy. Breast Cancer Res Treat 2012;133(2):659–66.

25. Prowler VL, Joh JE, Acs G, et al. Surgical excision of pure flat epithelial atypia identified on core needle breast biopsy. Breast 2014;23(4):352–6.

26. Lamb LR, Bahl M, Gadd MA, et al. Flat epithelial atypia: upgrade rates and risk-stratification approach to support informed decision making. J Am Coll Surg 2017;225(6):696–701.

27. Liu C, Dingee CK, Warburton R, et al. Pure flat epithelial atypia identified on core needle biopsy does not require excision. Eur J Surg Oncol 2020; 46(2):235–9.

28. Racz JM, Carter JM, Degnim AC. Lobular neoplasia and atypical ductal hyperplasia on core biopsy: current surgical management recommendations. Ann Surg Oncol 2017;24(10):2848–54.

29. King TA, Reis-Filho JS. Lobular neoplasia. Surg Oncol Clin N Am 2014;23(3):487–503.

30. Ginter PS, D'Alfonso TM. Current concepts in diagnosis, molecular features, and management of lobular carcinoma in situ of the breast with a discussion of morphologic variants. Arch Pathol Lab Med 2017;141(12):1668–78.

31. Maxwell AJ, Clements K, Dodwell DJ, et al. The radiological features, diagnosis and management of screen-detected lobular neoplasia of the breast: findings from the Sloane Project. Breast 2016;27: 109–15.

32. Wen HY, Brogi E. Lobular carcinoma in situ. Surg Pathol Clin 2018;11(1):123–45.

33. Khoury T, Kumar PR, Li Z, et al. Lobular neoplasia detected in MRI-guided core biopsy carries a high risk for upgrade: a study of 63 cases from four different institutions. Mod Pathol 2016;29(1):25–33.

34. Murray MP, Luedtke C, Liberman L, et al. Classic lobular carcinoma in situ and atypical lobular hyperplasia at percutaneous breast core biopsy: outcomes of prospective excision. Cancer 2013; 119(5):1073–9.

35. Nakhlis F, Gilmore L, Gelman R, et al. Incidence of adjacent synchronous invasive carcinoma and/or ductal carcinoma in-situ in patients with lobular neoplasia on core biopsy: results from a prospective multi-institutional registry (TBCRC 020). Ann Surg Oncol 2016;23(3):722–8.

36. Rendi MH, Dintzis SM, Lehman CD, et al. Lobular in-situ neoplasia on breast core needle biopsy: imaging indication and pathologic extent can identify which patients require excisional biopsy. Ann Surg Oncol 2012;19(3):914–21.

37. Wei S. Papillary Lesions of the breast: an update. Arch Pathol Lab Med 2016;140(7):628–43.

38. Krishnamurthy S, Bevers T, Kuerer H, et al. Multidisciplinary considerations in the management of high-risk breast lesions. AJR Am J Roentgenol 2012; 198(2):W132–40.

39. Wen X, Cheng W. Nonmalignant breast papillary lesions at core-needle biopsy: a meta-analysis of underestimation and influencing factors. Ann Surg Oncol 2013;20(1):94–101.

40. Bianchi S, Bendinelli B, Saladino V, et al. Non-malignant breast papillary lesions - b3 diagnosed on ultrasound–guided 14-gauge needle core biopsy: analysis of 114 cases from a single institution and review of the literature. Pathol Oncol Res 2015;21(3): 535–46.

41. Choi HY, Kim SM, Jang M, et al. Benign breast papilloma without atypia: outcomes of surgical excision versus US-guided directional vacuum-assisted removal or US follow-up. Radiology 2019;293(1): 72–80.

42. Ahn SK, Han W, Moon HG, et al. Management of benign papilloma without atypia diagnosed at ultrasound-guided core needle biopsy: scoring system for predicting malignancy. Eur J Surg Oncol 2018;44(1):53–8.

43. Symbol B, Ricci A Jr. Management of intraductal papilloma without atypia of the breast diagnosed on core biopsy: size and sampling matter. Breast J 2018;24(5):738–42.

44. Calhoun BC. Core needle biopsy of the breast: an evaluation of contemporary data. Surg Pathol Clin 2018;11(1):1–16.

45. Cohen MA, Newell MS. Radial scars of the breast encountered at core biopsy: review of histologic, imaging, and management considerations. AJR Am J Roentgenol 2017;209(5):1168–77.

46. Racz JM, Carter JM, Degnim AC. Challenging atypical breast lesions including flat epithelial atypia, radial scar, and intraductal papilloma. Ann Surg Oncol 2017;24(10):2842–7.

47. Linda A, Zuiani C, Furlan A, et al. Radial scars without atypia diagnosed at imaging-guided needle biopsy: how often is associated malignancy found at subsequent surgical excision, and do mammography and sonography predict which lesions are malignant? AJR Am J Roentgenol 2010;194(4): 1146–51.

48. Bahl M, Lamb LR, Lehman CD. Pathologic outcomes of architectural distortion on digital 2D versus tomosynthesis mammography. AJR Am J Roentgenol 2017;209(5):1162–7.

49. Farshid G, Buckley E. Meta-analysis of upgrade rates in 3163 radial scars excised after needle core biopsy diagnosis. Breast Cancer Res Treat 2019;174(1):165–77.

50. Andacoglu O, Kanbour-Shakir A, Teh YC, et al. Rationale of excisional biopsy after the diagnosis of benign radial scar on core biopsy: a single institutional outcome analysis. Am J Clin Oncol 2013; 36(1):7–11.

51. Miller CL, West JA, Bettini AC, et al. Surgical excision of radial scars diagnosed by core biopsy may help predict future risk of breast cancer. Breast Cancer Res Treat 2014;145(2):331–8.

52. Lamb LR, Bahl M, Hughes KS, et al. Pathologic upgrade rates of high-risk breast lesions on digital two-dimensional vs tomosynthesis mammography. J Am Coll Surg 2018;226(5):858–67.

53. Phantana-Angkool A, Forster MR, Warren YE, et al. Rate of radial scars by core biopsy and upgrading to malignancy or high-risk lesions before and after introduction of digital breast tomosynthesis. Breast Cancer Res Treat 2019;173(1):23–9.

54. Middleton LP, Sneige N, Coyne R, et al. Most lobular carcinoma in situ and atypical lobular hyperplasia diagnosed on core needle biopsy can be managed clinically with radiologic follow-up in a multidisciplinary setting. Cancer Med 2014;3(3):492–9.

55. Krishnamurthy S, Bevers T, Kuerer HM, et al. Paradigm shifts in breast care delivery: impact of imaging in a multidisciplinary environment. AJR Am J Roentgenol 2017;208(2):248–55.

56. Pediconi F, Padula S, Dominelli V, et al. Role of breast MR imaging for predicting malignancy of histologically borderline lesions diagnosed at core needle biopsy: prospective evaluation. Radiology 2010; 257(3):653–61.

57. Linda A, Zuiani C, Furlan A, et al. Nonsurgical management of high-risk lesions diagnosed at core needle biopsy: can malignancy be ruled out safely with breast MRI? AJR Am J Roentgenol 2012;198(2):272–80.

58. Londero V, Zuiani C, Linda A, et al. High-risk breast lesions at imaging-guided needle biopsy: usefulness of MRI for treatment decision. AJR Am J Roentgenol 2012;199(2):W240–50.

59. Bahl M, Barzilay R, Yedidia AB, et al. High-risk breast lesions: a machine learning model to

predict pathologic upgrade and reduce unnecessary surgical excision. Radiology 2018;286(3): 810–8.

60. NCCN Clinical Practice Guidelines in Oncology. Breast cancer risk reduction, version 1.2020. Available at: https://www.nccn.org/professionals/physician_gls/pdf/breast_risk.pdf. Accessed May 1, 2020.

61. Saslow D, Boetes C, Burke W, et al. American Cancer Society guidelines for breast screening with MRI as an adjunct to mammography. CA Cancer J Clin 2007;57(2):75–89.

62. Monticciolo DL, Newell MS, Moy L, et al. Breast cancer screening in women at higher-than-average risk: recommendations from the ACR. J Am Coll Radiol 2018;15(3 Pt A):408–14.

Understanding the Mammography Audit

Kimberly Funaro, MD[a,b,*], Dana Ataya, MD[a,b], Bethany Niell, MD, PhD[a,b]

KEYWORDS

• Mammography • Audit • Benchmarks • MQSA • Performance

KEY POINTS

- To be compliant with the Mammography Quality Standards Act, the US Food and Drug Administration mandates a medical outcomes audit program for each facility on an annual basis.
- The audit required by the US Food and Drug Administration differs from the audit recommendations from the American College of Radiology.
- Separate audit data should be collected for screening mammograms and diagnostic mammograms because the performance benchmarks differ.
- To gauge performance, use multiple audit metrics rather than a single metric.
- Double reading, increasing reading volumes, obtaining all available prior examinations, reviewing call backs, and reviewing false-negative cases may improve performance.

INTRODUCTION

Mammography remains the gold standard for breast cancer screening and has been proven to reduce breast cancer mortality; however, there is variability in the performance of mammography across different facilities and radiologists.[1–4] To establish uniform quality standards, the Mammography Quality Standards Act (MQSA) was enacted in 1992.[5] The US Food and Drug Administration (FDA) issued the MQSA final regulations, under which mammography facilities are currently regulated.[6] The MQSA requires each mammography facility to meet certain quality standards, maintain certification and accreditation, and undergo regular inspections and surveys.[7]

As a part of the quality assurance process, a medical outcomes audit is required at least once every 12 months at each mammography facility.[7] Per the MQSA, there should be a system in place to track "positive" mammograms, collect pathology results from biopsies performed, correlate the pathology results with the final assessment category, review any known false-negative mammograms, and assess medical outcomes audit data.[7,8] At a minimum, facilities must track "positive" mammograms interpreted as suspicious or highly suggestive of malignancy. Individual as well as aggregate performance parameters should be calculated and a designated interpreting physician, known as the lead interpreting physician, should review the data and be responsible for documenting audit results and notifying the other radiologists of their results.[7]

The American College of Radiology (ACR) asserts that more complex auditing than required by MQSA should be performed to determine acceptable clinical performance.[8] The ACR has published the procedures for performing a basic and more complete audit in the Breast Imaging Reporting and Data Systems (BI-RADS) Atlas.[8] The audit allows assessment of strengths and weaknesses when compared with nationally recognized benchmarks.[4,9–11]

This article defines the ACR mammography audit terminology, reviews the basic and more

[a] Department of Diagnostic Imaging and Interventional Radiology, H. Lee Moffitt Cancer Center, 12902 USF Magnolia Drive, Tampa, FL 33612, USA; [b] Department of Oncologic Sciences, University of South Florida, H. Lee Moffitt Cancer Center and Research Institute, Tampa, FL, USA
* Corresponding author. H. Lee Moffitt Cancer Center and Research Institute, 12902 USF Magnolia Drive, Tampa, FL 33612.
E-mail address: kimberly.funaro@moffitt.org

Radiol Clin N Am 59 (2021) 41–55
https://doi.org/10.1016/j.rcl.2020.09.009
0033-8389/21/© 2020 Elsevier Inc. All rights reserved.

complete mammography audit, and discusses how to assess your practice and individual performance relative to published performance benchmarks.

AUDIT TERMS AND DEFINITIONS

This section reviews the basic audit terminology and provides pertinent examples.

Screening Mammography Versus Diagnostic Mammography

Positive screening examination
Additional diagnostic imaging is recommended or a tissue diagnosis[a] is recommended. BI-RADS assessments of 3, 4, or 5 at screening are highly discouraged (Box 1) (Table 1).[8] Note that a positive screening mammogram as defined by the ACR is different than the definition of a positive examination in the MQSA Final Rule.[8]

Positive diagnostic examination
Tissue diagnosis is recommended (see Table 1).

Negative screening examination
An examination evaluated as negative or benign (BI-RADS 1 or 2).

Negative diagnostic examination
A tissue diagnosis was not recommended. The examination was assessed as negative (BI-RADS 1), benign (BI-RADS 2) or probably benign (BI-RADS 3[b]).

Cancer
Defined as a tissue diagnosis of ductal carcinoma in situ or any type of primary invasive breast carcinoma (Table 2).[8] Table 2 also includes a subset of the pathology results that are not included in the definition of cancer for the purposes of the audit.

Box 1
Screening versus diagnostic

Screening mammogram

> Performed to detect occult breast cancer in asymptomatic patients

Diagnostic mammogram

> Indications include
>
> i. Call back after screening mammogram
>
> ii. Clinical signs or symptoms
>
> iii. Follow-up imaging of a probably benign finding
>
> iv. Response evaluation after neoadjuvant treatment for breast cancer

Asymptomatic women with a personal history of breast cancer or benign biopsy may undergo annual diagnostic rather than screening mammograms. For audit purposes, those examinations should be included in the screening group.

Coding of Mammograms

True positive
A true-positive result is a tissue diagnosis of cancer within 1 year after a positive examination (Figs. 1–3, Tables 3 and 4). Remember, a positive screening mammogram is defined differently than a positive diagnostic mammogram (Box 2).

False positive
A false-positive result is no known tissue diagnosis of breast cancer within 1 year of a positive examination (Boxes 3 and 4). For auditing purposes, 3 separate definitions exist and are outlined in detail in the BI-RADS Atlas.[8]

Table 1
Positive screening and diagnostic assessments

Positive Screening Examination	Positive Diagnostic Examination
BI-RADS 0	BI-RADS 0 [b]
BI-RADS 3, 4, 5[a]	BI-RADS 4 and 5

[a] Use of BI-RADS 3, 4, and 5 on a screening mammogram is *highly discouraged*.
[b] Use of BI-RADS 0 at diagnostic mammography is *discouraged*. An addendum issuing a final assessment should be performed. For the rare instance in which a BI-RADS 0 assessment remains for a diagnostic mammogram, the examination is coded positive.

---

[a]*Tissue diagnosis.* Pathologic diagnosis made by an interventional procedure (fine-needle aspiration, core biopsy, or incisional or excisional biopsy).[8]

[b]A BI-RADS 3 assessment is coded as negative for diagnostic mammography, but positive for screening mammography.

Table 2
Cancer versus not cancer

Cancer (Breast Cancer)	Not Breast Cancer
Invasive ductal carcinoma Invasive lobular carcinoma Ductal carcinoma in situ	Metastatic cancers to the breast (ie, not breast origin) Lymphoma/leukemia Malignant phyllodes tumor Breast sarcoma Lobular carcinoma in situ Atypical ductal hyperplasia Atypical lobular hyperplasia

True negative

A true-negative result is defined as no known tissue diagnosis of breast cancer within 1 year of a negative examination (see **Box 4**).

False negative

A false-negative result is defined as a tissue diagnosis of cancer within 1 year of a negative examination (**Box 5**).

Interval cancer

An interval cancer is a cancer that is diagnosed within 1 year of a negative examination.

Positive Predictive Value

Three separate definitions exist of a positive predictive values (PPV).[8]

i. PPV_1: Abnormal findings at screening (**Box 6**).
ii. PPV_2: Biopsy recommended. PPV_2 is a metric intended to assess diagnostic mammograms (**Box 7**).

iii. PPV_3: Biopsy performed or biopsy yield of malignancy or positive biopsy rate. PPV_3 is a measure designed to assess diagnostic mammograms (**Box 8**).

Sensitivity

The sensitivity is the probability of a positive examination when cancer exists (**Box 9**).

Specificity

The specificity is the probability of a negative examination when cancer does not exist (**Box 10**). Sensitivity and specificity are only measured with sufficient accuracy if outcomes data are linked to a tumor registry. Therefore, many practices cannot calculate sensitivity and specificity in their audit report.[8]

Cancer Detection Rate

The cancer detection rate is the number of cancers identified at imaging per 1000 examinations

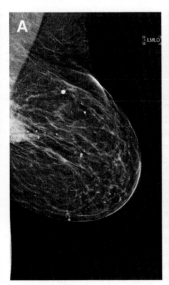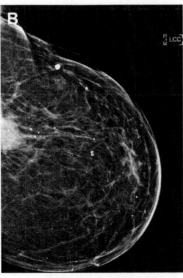

Fig. 1. Left mediolateral oblique (*A*) and craniocaudal (*B*) diagnostic mammogram images demonstrate a suspicious mass (BI-RADS 4) in the posterior central left breast. Ultrasound-guided biopsy yielded leiomyosarcoma; therefore, the diagnostic mammogram was coded as a false positive.

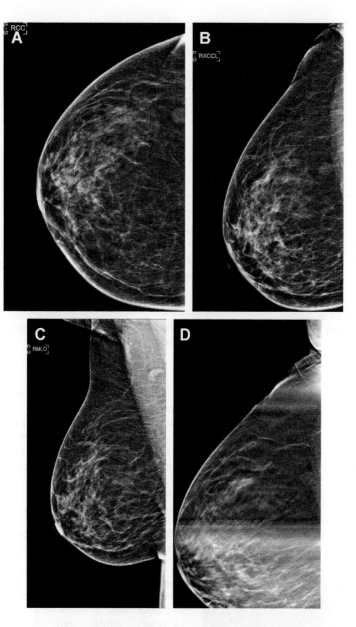

Fig. 2. Right craniocaudal (*A*), exaggerated craniocaudal (*B*), and mediolateral oblique (*C*) baseline screening mammogram images demonstrate a mass in the lateral right breast (reported as BI-RADS 0). Tomosynthesis spot compression view (*D*) demonstrates the mass to be oval and circumscribed. Ultrasound examination (not shown) demonstrated an oval and circumscribed hypoechoic mass. A BI-RADS 3 assessment was given. Two years of follow-up demonstrated stability of the finding and it was then downgraded to a BI-RADS 2. Therefore, the screening mammogram is coded false positive and the diagnostic mammogram as a true negative.

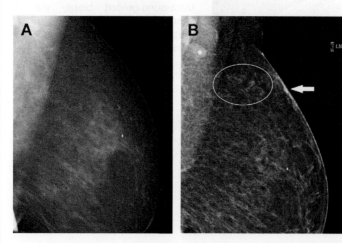

Fig. 3. Left mediolateral oblique (*A*) screening mammogram (reported as BI-RADS 1) and left mediolateral oblique diagnostic mammogram (*B*) were performed 5 months apart. The patient developed skin changes (*arrow*) and clinical axillary adenopathy (*star*), prompting diagnostic mammogram. A new asymmetry (*circle*) is present on the mediolateral oblique view (BI-RADS 4). Image guided biopsy demonstrated lymphoma; therefore, the diagnostic mammogram is coded as a false positive and the screening mammogram as a true negative.

Table 3
Biopsy results – screening

	Biopsy Results	
	Positive (Tissue Diagnosis of Cancer Within 1 Year)	Negative (Benign Concordant Tissue Diagnosis, or No Tissue Diagnosis of Cancer Within 1 Year)
Positive screening mammogram (BI-RADS 0, 3, 4, 5)	True positive	False positive
Negative screening mammogram (BI-RADS 1, 2)	False negative	True negative

Adapted from Sickles, E., D'Orsi CJ, ACR BI-RADS® Follow-up and Outcome Monitoring. In: ACR BI-RADS® Atlas, Breast Imaging Reporting and Data System. 2013, Reston, VA: American College of Radiology; with permission.

performed. This metric should be calculated separately for screening and diagnostic examinations. In the screening setting, the cancer detection rate should be calculated separately for prevalent cancers (those found at the first round of screening) and for incident cancers (those found at subsequent screening).[8]

Abnormal Interpretation Rate

The abnormal interpretation rate is the percentage of examinations interpreted as positive (see **Table 1**). Calculation of the recall rate adds value only if it represents all positive screening mammograms (BI-RADS 0, 3, 4, or 5) and is therefore equivalent to the abnormal interpretation rate.[8] If screening mammograms are only assessed BI-RADS categories 0, 1, or 2, as recommended by the BI-RADS Atlas, the recall rate and the abnormal interpretation rate will both reflect the percentage of screening mammograms recommended for recall.

THE BASIC CLINICALLY RELEVANT MAMMOGRAPHY AUDIT

The mammography audit allows individuals and practices to measure outcomes and assess if they are meeting the major goals of breast cancer screening: (1) finding a high percentage of cancers that exist in asymptomatic women undergoing screening (measured with cancer detection rate), (2) finding those cancers with an acceptable range of recommendations for additional imaging and biopsies (measured with abnormal interpretation rate and PPV), and (3) finding a high percentage of small, node negative, early stage cancers that are more likely curable (measured with percentage of "minimal," node-negative, and stage 0 or 1 cancers).[8,12]

Table 4
Biopsy results – diagnostic

	Biopsy Results	
	Positive (Tissue Diagnosis of Cancer Within 1 Year)	Negative (Benign Concordant Tissue Diagnosis, or No Tissue Diagnosis of Cancer Within 1 Year)
Positive diagnostic mammogram (BI-RADS 4, 5)[a]	True positive	False positive
Negative diagnostic mammogram (BI-RADS 1, 2, 3)	False negative	True negative

[a] Use of BI-RADS 0 at diagnostic mammography is *discouraged*. An addendum issuing a final assessment should be performed. For the rare instance in which a BI-RADS 0 assessment remains for a diagnostic mammogram, the examination is coded positive.

Adapted from Sickles, E., D'Orsi CJ, ACR BI-RADS® Follow-up and Outcome Monitoring. In: ACR BI-RADS® Atlas, Breast Imaging Reporting and Data System. 2013, Reston, VA: American College of Radiology; with permission.

> **Box 2**
> **True-positive example**
>
> A woman is recalled from screening for additional imaging (BI-RADS 0). The diagnostic mammogram is suspicious (BI-RADS 4) with a recommendation for tissue sampling. Biopsy yields a breast malignancy. Both the screening and diagnostic examinations are positive and breast cancer is diagnosed within 1 year—therefore, both examinations are classified as true positives.

> **Box 4**
> **BI-RADS category 3 example (false positive and true negative)**
>
> A woman is recalled from baseline screening for additional imaging (BI-RADS 0). On diagnostic mammography, an oval circumscribed mass is assessed BI-RADS 3 (see **Fig. 2**). No breast cancer is diagnosed within 1 year of the examination. The screening mammogram is coded as a false positive, and the diagnostic mammogram is coded as a true negative.

Federal regulations specify that a facility's first audit must be initiated no later than 12 months after certification, and the audit must be completed within an additional 12 months.[7] The additional 12 months are required to collect pathology data and allow time for determination of cancer status.[7,8]

The MQSA requires a facility to have a method to follow-up with all positive mammograms and a system to collect pathology results and to correlate the pathology and mammography results, as well as the mandate to review any known false negatives occurring within 12 months of mammography.[7] However, best practices outlined by the BI-RADS Atlas recommend certain minimum raw data be collected and used to calculate derived data, both of which are steps beyond the federal regulations, to allow for a more clinically relevant measurement of practice and individual outcomes (**Table 5**).[8]

THE MORE COMPLETE AUDIT

The basic clinically relevant mammography audit provides essential data to assess the performance of mammography interpretations. However, additional data may be collected and derived to provide further information on mammographic performance, known as the more complete audit (**Boxes 11** and **12**).[8] In particular, the more complete audit provides practices with in-depth data

regarding their patient risk factors, imaging characteristics of cancers detected, and the incidence versus prevalence cancer detection rate, which are not assessed with a basic audit.

The more complete audit also recommends that derived data in the basic audit be calculated separately for screening mammograms as well as subtypes of diagnostic examinations (eg, recall from screening mammography, short-term follow-up, or a further evaluation of a palpable lump).[8] As with the basic clinically relevant mammography audit, the calculation of multiple metrics provides the most useful information. Accurate ascertainment of true negatives, true positives, false positives, and false negatives will be difficult if the practice is not linked to a regional tumor registry or in a tumor registry of a large organization with a nonmobile patient population.[8] These limitations should be acknowledged when calculating audit data.

WHAT IS MY MAMMOGRAPHY AUDIT TELLING ME?

Radiologists have difficulty accurately gauging their interpretive performance. More than 70% of radiologists can accurately estimate their cancer detection rate and recall rate, but the remainder tended to underestimate the recall rate and overestimate the cancer detection rate.[13] Only 25% can accurately estimate the PPV_2, despite 96% reporting that they have previously received their

> **Box 3**
> **False-positive example**
>
> Diagnostic mammography is performed for a new, palpable lump in the left breast (see **Fig. 1**). A suspicious mass is present, and biopsy is recommended (BI-RADS 4). Biopsy yields leiomyosarcoma. The diagnostic mammogram (BI-RADS 4) is classified as false positive because no breast malignancy is diagnosed within 1 year.

> **Box 5**
> **False-negative example**
>
> Screening mammography was assigned BI-RADS 2. Patient presents 6 months later with a palpable mass, which is biopsied and yields cancer. The screening examination was interpreted as negative, but malignancy is diagnosed within 1 year, therefore the screening examination is a false negative.

audit reports.[13] Because radiologists tend to perceive their performance as better than it actually is, radiologists who interpret mammography must understand their audit results so that they can address any performance gaps.

Most radiologists consider audits valuable and use them to review performance and false negatives.[14] Baseline low performers show the most benefit from audit feedback.[15,16] The audit and feedback are most effective when delivered by a supervisor with both verbal and written components that include explicit targets and an action plan.[15,16]

For the audit data to be the most useful, outcomes for the facility as well as individual radiologists should be compared with standard performance benchmarks (Box 13). Per the BI-RADS Atlas, the mammographic audit data may be compared with (1) recommendations from an expert panel of breast imaging interpreting physicians based on analysis of published data and extensive personal experience; (2) benchmarks reported by the Breast Cancer Surveillance Consortium (BCSC); or (3) outcomes reported from the ACR National Mammography Database (NMD).[8] Benchmarks differ for screening versus diagnostic mammography, so it is critical to collect and calculate them separately.[4,8,17]

Expert Panel Benchmarks for Mammography

The expert panels consisted of 10 radiologists for the screening portion and 11 radiologists for the diagnostic portion, with a mixture from academic institutions as well as community practices.[17,18] Performance ranges in both studies, screening and diagnostic mammography, used a modified Angoff approach in which a panel of judges determined a minimally acceptable level of performance.[17,18] The panels drafted their cut points for performance, understanding that individual radiologists falling below standards might be recommended for additional training (Table 6).

Breast Cancer Surveillance Consortium Benchmarks for Mammography

Over the past 2 decades, the BCSC has collected data from a collaborative group of 6 active breast imaging registries and 2 historic registries from different geographic regions across the United States, with more than 90% collected from nonacademic community-based imaging facilities.[10,19] Each registry is linked to a state tumor registry or to the Surveillance Epidemiology and End Results program to ensure near complete cancer ascertainment.[10,20] Audit data are collected and calculated, and additional information on clinical outcomes, patient demographics, and clinical information are compiled (Table 7).

Audit benchmarks in the BI-RADS Atlas 5th edition and Table 7 are BCSC data from 1996 to 2005, compiled from more than 4 million screening mammograms, more than 400,000 diagnostic mammograms, more than 150 mammography facilities, and more than 700 interpreting radiologists.[8] To address the transition from screen film mammography to digital mammography in the United States, the BCSC compiled data from more than 90 mammography facilities and more than 350 individual radiologists between 2007 and 2013. Updated performance benchmarks from more than 1.6 million digital screening mammograms and 400,000 digital diagnostic mammograms are presented in Table 8.[9,19]

In the BCSC, digital screening mammography demonstrated an increased sensitivity of 87% compared with 79% for screen film mammography, likely secondary to the improved performance of digital mammography in younger women and women with dense breasts.[9,21] More than 90% of radiologists achieved the recommended ranges for sensitivity and cancer detection rate. However, almost one-half of the interpreting radiologists had abnormal interpretation rates that were higher than the recommended rate.[9]

Although the performance measures in Table 8 are averaged across all diagnostic indications, it is important to remember that measures vary by diagnostic indication. For example, women undergoing diagnostic mammography for a palpable lump are much more likely to have a positive mammogram, biopsy recommendation, and cancer diagnosis compared with women undergoing short interval follow-up imaging or additional evaluation of a screening mammogram finding.[19] The cancer detection rate for a palpable lump for the updated BCSC data was 64.5 per 1000 with PPV_2 of 34.5%, PPV_3 of 37.7%, and sensitivity of 92.3%.[19] Compared with screen film diagnostic mammography, digital diagnostic mammography demonstrated higher abnormal interpretation rates and cancer detection rates, but decreased PPVs.[19] Less than 70% of radiologists were within the acceptable range for PPV_2, PPV_3, or specificity, suggesting that there is room for

improvement in the decrease of false-positive biopsy recommendations.[19]

American College of Radiology National Mammography Database Benchmarks

The NMD was established in 2008 and is a component of the ACR National Radiology Data Registry.[22,23] It was designed as a quality improvement tool so mammography facilities could compare their performance metrics with local, regional, and national peer facilities.[11] The NMD collects self-reported data on the mammography facility characteristics. Patient demographics are self-reported from patient screening questionnaires, and data from the mammographic image interpretation are also compiled.[11] The NMD relies on facility-reported pathology outcomes, rather than linkage to tumor registries. Using data from more than 3.1 million screening mammograms and 90 facilities between 2008 and 2012, the NMD calculated facility-level performance measures (Table 9). Note that these NMD measures are at the facility level, whereas the BCSC reports at the interpreting radiologist level.

Table 5
Data for the basic mammography audit

Data to be Collected	Derived Data to be Calculated
1. Dates of audit period and total number of examinations in that period 2. Numbers of screening and diagnostic mammograms[a] 3. Number of screening mammogram recalls (BI-RADS 0) 4. Number of short-interval follow-up examinations (BI-RADS 3) 5. Number of recommendations for tissue diagnosis (BI-RADS 4, 5) 6. Tissue diagnosis results: malignant or benign 7. Cancer staging: histologic type, invasive cancer size, nodal status, and tumor grade 8. Analysis of any known false-negative mammography examinations (required per MQSA final rule)	1. True positive 2. False positives (FP_1, FP_2, FP_3) 3. Positive predictive value (PPV_1, PPV_2, PPV_3) 4. Cancer detection rate 5. Percentage of node-negative invasive cancers 6. Percentage of "minimal" cancers (invasive cancer ≤ 1 cm or ductal carcinoma in situ) 7. Percentage of stage 0 or 1 cancers 8. Abnormal interpretation (recall) rate for screening mammograms

[a] Separate audit statistics should be maintained for screening and diagnostic examinations.
Adapted from Sickles, E., D'Orsi CJ, ACR BI-RADS® Follow-up and Outcome Monitoring. In: ACR BI-RADS® Atlas, Breast Imaging Reporting and Data System. 2013, Reston, VA: American College of Radiology.

During the study time frame, the recall rate and cancer detection rate decreased, whereas the PPV$_2$ increased.[11] NMD data regarding breast cancer size, tumor stage, and nodal involvement have not yet been published.

Applicability of the Benchmarks and Use in Practice

The BI-RADS Atlas provides the framework for how to perform the mammography audit and benchmarks provide reference for comparison of the audit data. But how should an individual radiologist and a mammography practice interpret their audit data?

Because the BCSC requires linkage to tumor registry data, the BCSC has near complete cancer ascertainment and can accurately calculate audit measures. Facilities without linkage to tumor registry data will (1) underascertain their true-positive examinations, thus having lower cancer detection rates and PPVs compared with BCSC benchmarks and (2) be unable to accurately calculate sensitivity and specificity.[8,24] The recall rate is the only widely used audit metric not impacted by accurate cancer ascertainment. Therefore, many mammography facilities in the United States will not be able to achieve benchmarks reported by the BCSC, with the exception of recall rate, unless they decide to link to a state or regional tumor registry.[24]

The NMD has rapidly increasing annual accrual over the past several years, with data from more than 12 million screening mammograms and 200 facilities by the end of 2016.[24] Participating mammography practices report data directly to the NMD. Because no on-site audits are performed, the NMD relies on facilities to accurately calculate audit measures and correct errors, if they exist.[25] The NMD provides performance reports to participating facilities every 6 months, allowing each facility to monitor temporal trends and compare their performance with peer facilities. The NMD has similar facility and patient demographic characteristics to the BCSC.[11] However, NMD facilities are impacted by the

Table 6
Expert panel benchmarks per the BI-RADS atlas

Expert Panel Benchmarks per the BI-RADS Atlas[17,18]			
	Screening	Diagnostic: Abnormal Screening	Diagnostic: Palpable Lump
Cancer detection rate	≥2.5	≥20	≥40
Abnormal interpretation (recall) rate	5%–12%	8%–25%	10%–25%
PPV_1	3%–8%	N/A	N/A
PPV_2	20%–40%	15%–40%	25%–50%
PPV_3	N/A	20%–45%	30%–55%
Sensitivity[a]	≥75%	≥80%	≥85%
Specificity[a]	88%–95%	80%–95%	83%–95%

Abbreviation: N/A, not applicable.
[a] Accurately measured only if data are linked to a tumor registry.
Data from Sickles, E., D'Orsi CJ, *ACR BI-RADS® Follow-up and Outcome Monitoring. In: ACR BI-RADS® Atlas, Breast Imaging Reporting and Data System.* 2013, Reston, VA: American College of Radiology.

same limitations of cancer underascertainment that affects nearly all practices in the United States. As a result, the argument has been made that NMD benchmarks may more closely reflect the average mammography practice and interpreting radiologist in the United States, compared with the BCSC.[11,24,25]

There has been a paradigm shift in health care payment reform to reward quality. In 2006, the Centers for Medicare and Medicaid Services adopted the mammography recall rate as 1 imaging efficiency performance measure.[26] The NMD is approved as a Qualified Clinical Data Registry for the Centers for Medicare and Medicaid Services

Table 7
BCSC mammography benchmarks per the BI-RADS atlas

BCSC Mammography Benchmarks per the BI-RADS Atlas[4,10]			
	Screening	Diagnostic: All Indications	Diagnostic: Palpable Lump
Cancer detection rate	4.7	30.0	57.7
Median size of invasive cancers (mm)	14.0	17.0	21.8
Percentage node negative invasive cancers	77.3%	68.2%	56.5%
Percentage minimal cancer	52.6%	39.8%	15.2%
Percentage stage 0 or 1 cancer	74.8%	60.7%	37%
Abnormal interpretation (recall) rate	10.6%	9.6%	13.3%
PPV_1	4.4%	N/A	N/A
PPV_2	25.4%	31.2%	43.7%
PPV_3	31%	35.9%	49.1%
Sensitivity[a]	79%	83.1%	87.8%
Specificity[a]	89.8%	93.2%	92.2%

Abbreviation: N/A, not applicable.
[a] Accurately measured only if data are linked to a tumor registry.
Data from Sickles, E., D'Orsi CJ, ACR BI-RADS® Follow-up and Outcome Monitoring. In: ACR BI-RADS® Atlas, Breast Imaging Reporting and Data System. 2013, Reston, VA: American College of Radiology.

Table 8
BCSC performance measures for digital mammography

BCSC Performance Measures for Digital Mammography[9,19]		
	Screening	Diagnostic: All Indications
Cancer detection rate	5.1	34.7
Abnormal interpretation (recall) rate	11.6%	12.6%
PPV_1	4.4%	N/A
PPV_2	25.6%	27.5%
PPV_3	28.6%	30.4%
Sensitivity[a]	86.9%	87.8%
Specificity[a]	88.9%	90.5%
Cancers stage 0 or 1	76.9%	63.4%
Minimal cancers	57.7%	45.6%

Abbreviation: N/A, not applicable.
  [a] Accurately measured only if data are linked to a tumor registry.

Physician Quality Reporting System.[26] Ideally, measures that are performance based and impact reimbursement should be within control of the group being measured and incentivized. It is increasingly important that radiologists who interpret mammograms understand how performance measures are calculated and what factors impact each metric. For the recall rate, the BI-RADS Atlas expert panel recommends a target of 5% to 12%, whereas the Agency for Healthcare Research and Quality has previously recommended 10%.[27] However, fewer than 60% of BCSC radiologists performed within the ACR-recommended range.[9] Numerous factors have been shown to impact the recall rate, including annual volume, batch and double reading, years of experience, and fellowship training.[28,29] For radiologists with too many false-positive screening examinations (a high recall rate outside of benchmark standards but a cancer detection rate that just meets the benchmark) strategies such as double reading when considering a call back and procuring all available priors may mitigate false positives in the future.[30,31]

The PPV measures the likelihood that a positive mammogram indicates the presence of breast cancer. The PPV_1 measures the effectiveness of screening interpretations, by incorporating both recall rate and cancer detection rate. Because the PPV_2 measures biopsies recommended, it is a useful metric of mammographic recommendations at the radiologist and facility levels.[24,25] For example, a PPV_2 substantially higher than published benchmarks indicates a high number of true positives in those studies recommended for biopsy, which may be a sign of poor performance because only lesions with a high likelihood of being cancer are recommended for biopsy, so smaller and more subtle malignancies may be getting missed.[24] Unlike the PPV_2, the PPV_3 incorporates

Table 9
NMD performance measures for screening mammography 2008–2012

NMD Performance Measures for Screening Mammography Between 2008 and 2012[11]		
	Mean	Interquartile Range (25th–75th Percentile)
Cancer detection rate	3.4	2.7–4.4
Abnormal interpretation (recall) rate	10%	7.8%–11.9%
PPV_2	18.5%	13.3%–23.3%
PPV_3	29.2%	21.4%–35.5%

Table 10 Acceptable ranges of radiologist performance[29]			
Criteria	Recall Rate (%)	Cancer Detection Rate per 1000	PPV$_1$ (%)
A	5–12	2.5–<4	3–8
B	3–15	≥4–<6	≥3
C	3–20	≥6	N/A

Abbreviation: N/A, not applicable.

Data from Miglioretti DL, Ichikawa L, Smith RA, et al. Criteria for identifying radiologists with acceptable screening mammography interpretive performance on basis of multiple performance measures. *AJR Am J Roentgenol.* 2015;204(4):W486 to 491.

biopsies actually performed. Using NMD and BCSC data, only 64% to 71% of recommended biopsies were reportedly performed.[11] This may be artificially low for the NMD at 64%, because they do not have tumor registry linkage and patients may have gone elsewhere for biopsy.[11] The PPV$_3$ is more useful at the societal level because it reflects whether the recommended clinical care was actually performed. The Institute of Medicine therefore supports the use of the PPV$_2$ rather than the PPV$_3$ as an indicator of quality performance.[24,25]

Because performance measures are interrelated, the interpretation of a single audit metric is not a useful measurement of performance.[8] An integrated assessment of the cancer detection rate, PPV, and recall rate yields greater value. To better illustrate how multiple metrics are useful for analysis, imagine an interpreting radiologist with a recall rate lower than the expert panel benchmark from the BI-RADS Atlas (<5%). If the same radiologist's cancer detection rate is low (<2 per 1000), this result may indicate poor performance, and the radiologist's performance should be reviewed within the context of their individual practice to determine whether additional training should be considered. Conversely, if that same radiologist had an above average cancer detection rate combined with the low recall rate, that would indicate optimal performance. For individual readers and practices who interpret low volumes of screening mammograms, it will be difficult to gauge an accurate cancer detection rate given the low prevalence of cancers in the screening population.[8,24] In those situations, auditing cumulative data over more than 1 year may be necessary to obtain a more accurate cancer detection rate.[8]

To identify radiologists with an acceptable screening mammogram interpretative performance, an expert panel created performance criteria based on multiple audit measures.[29] For facilities with linkage to tumor registry data, the panel recommended that radiologists with sensitivity of 80% or greater have a specificity of 85% or greater, whereas lower sensitivity (75%–79%) would require higher specificity (88%–97%).[29] For facilities without tumor registry linkage, the panel issued 3 different sets of combined criteria for acceptable ranges of recall rates, cancer detection rate, and PPV$_1$ that are broken down as criteria A, B, and C in **Table 10**.[29] For criterion C, the PPV$_1$ must be 3% or greater to achieve a cancer detection rate and recall rate within those ranges, so the PPV$_1$ does not require consideration in this group. Only 60% of radiologists who interpreted more than 1000 screening mammograms within the BCSC met any of these 3 criteria.[29]

Additional Considerations

The effect of annual mammography volumes on reader performance must be considered when evaluating audit results. Cancer detection rates and PPV in any given year should be interpreted with caution for low-volume practices and low-volume readers.[8,24] In that situation, annual audits with 2 or more years of cumulative data would provide more meaningful data.[8] Additionally, many practices have shifted from digital mammography to combination mammography with digital breast tomosynthesis or digital breast tomosynthesis alone with a synthesized 2-dimensional mammogram. Because digital breast tomosynthesis has been shown to decrease recall rate with a slight incremental increase in cancer detection rate, practices incorporating tomosynthesis should remain cognizant of these potential changes in performance when interpreting their audit metrics and comparing them with published benchmarks for film screen or full-field digital mammography examinations.[32,33]

Within the United States, to meet continuing experience requirements, radiologists must interpret 960 mammograms every 2 years.[7] By comparison, 3000 to 5000 mammograms per year are required or recommended in European screening programs, which have lower recall rates and similar cancer detection rates.[34–36] The relationship between mammography volume and interpretive performance is complex and multifactorial.[11,37] A higher volume tends to be associated with a lower recall rate and false positives without a loss of cancer detection rate or sensitivity.[37] Radiologists with a greater screening focus have been found to have lower sensitivities and cancer detection rates and significantly lower false-positive rates.[37,38] Radiologists with low diagnostic mammography volumes tend to have lower cancer detection rates for screening mammography.[37] Therefore, increasing the minimum screening volume requirement and adding a minimal volume requirement for diagnostic mammography interpretation may improve the quality of screening mammography in the United States.[36–38]

Reader characteristics and experience also play a role in interpreting audit results. Higher recall and false-positive rates occur in readers with less than 10 years of experience and in readers who have interpreted fewer than 20,000 cumulative mammograms.[3,36] Additionally, fellowship training in breast imaging is significantly associated with greater sensitivity and accuracy, but also higher false-positive rates.[3]

There are important differences in the performance of mammography in the United States compared with other countries. The United States performs screening mammography at a younger age and at more frequent intervals than in countries with government-funded health care and screening programs.[24,39,40] Screening annually, rather than every 2 to 3 years, produces different audit outcomes. In addition, suggested recall rates in the United States reported by both the BCSC and NMD are higher than the recommended United Kingdom (5%–7%) and European guidelines (<5%) and should not be used as benchmarks outside of the United States.[4,26] There has also been less emphasis on reducing false positives in the United States.[24]

SUMMARY

The mammography audit is a critical tool allowing individual radiologists and practices to gauge their performance against published benchmarks to address performance gaps and maximize the utility of screening mammography—finding the most cancers at the smallest and most treatable stage, while maintaining an acceptable false-positive rate.

CLINICS CARE POINTS

- A BIRADS 3 assessment on diagnostic mammography is coded as a negative diagnostic examination.
- "Cancer" per the mammography audit is only defined as only a primary breast cancer (in situ or invasive).
- In the United States, radiologists must interpret 960 mammograms every 2 years to meet continuing experience requirements by the MQSA.
- Sensitivity and specificity are difficult for practices to accurately calculate unless linked to a tumor registry (which allows near complete cancer ascertainment).

DISCLOSURE

The authors have no disclosures or conflicts of interests.

REFERENCES

1. Tabar L, Fagerberg CJ, Gad A, et al. Reduction in mortality from breast cancer after mass screening with mammography. Randomised trial from the Breast Cancer Screening Working Group of the Swedish National Board of Health and Welfare. Lancet 1985;1(8433):829–32.
2. Smith RA, Duffy SW, Gabe R, et al. The randomized trials of breast cancer screening: what have we learned? Radiol Clin North Am 2004;42(5):793–806.
3. Elmore JG, Jackson SL, Abraham L, et al. Variability in interpretive performance at screening mammography and radiologists' characteristics associated with accuracy. Radiology 2009;253(3):641–51.
4. Rosenberg RD, Yankaskas BC, Abraham LA, et al. Performance benchmarks for screening mammography. Radiology 2006;241(1):55–66.
5. Monsees BS. The Mammography Quality Standards Act. An overview of the regulations and guidance. Radiol Clin North Am 2000;38(4):759–72.
6. U.S. Food and Drug Administration. The Mammography Quality Standards Act final regulations: preparing for MQSA inspections; final guidance for industry and FDA. Document issued November 5. 2001. Available at: https://www.fda.gov/media/74027/download. Accessed April 14, 2020.
7. Mammography Quality Standards Act Regulations. U.S. Food & Drug Administration. Available at: https://www.fda.gov/radiation-emitting-products/regulations-mqsa/mammography-quality-standards-act-regulations#s90012. Accessed March 2, 2020.
8. Sickles E, D'Orsi CJ. ACR BI-RADS® follow-up and outcome monitoring. In: D'Orsi CJ, editor. ACR BI-RADS® atlas, breast imaging reporting and data

system. Reston (VA): American College of Radiology; 2013. p. 5-67.

9. Lehman CD, Arao RF, Sprague BL, et al. National performance benchmarks for modern screening digital mammography: update from the Breast Cancer Surveillance Consortium. Radiology 2017; 283(1):49–58.

10. Sickles EA, Miglioretti DL, Ballard-Barbash R, et al. Performance benchmarks for diagnostic mammography. Radiology 2005;235(3):775–90.

11. Lee CS, Bhargavan-Chatfield M, Burnside ES, et al. The National Mammography Database: preliminary data. AJR Am J Roentgenol 2016;206(4): 883–90.

12. Linver MN, Osuch JR, Brenner RJ, et al. The mammography audit: a primer for the mammography quality standards act (MQSA). AJR Am J Roentgenol 1995;165(1):19–25.

13. Cook AJ, Elmore JG, Zhu W, et al. Mammographic interpretation: radiologists' ability to accurately estimate their performance and compare it with that of their peers. AJR Am J Roentgenol 2012;199(3): 695–702.

14. Elmore JG, Aiello Bowles EJ, Geller B, et al. Radiologists' attitudes and use of mammography audit reports. Acad Radiol 2010;17(6):752–60.

15. Jamtvedt G, Young JM, Kristoffersen DT, et al. Does telling people what they have been doing change what they do? A systematic review of the effects of audit and feedback. Qual Saf Health Care 2006; 15(6):433–6.

16. Ivers N, Jamtvedt G, Flottorp S, et al. Audit and feedback: effects on professional practice and healthcare outcomes. Cochrane Database Syst Rev 2012;(6):Cd000259.

17. Carney PA, Parikh J, Sickles EA, et al. Diagnostic mammography: identifying minimally acceptable interpretive performance criteria. Radiology 2013; 267(2):359–67.

18. Carney PA, Sickles EA, Monsees BS, et al. Identifying minimally acceptable interpretive performance criteria for screening mammography. Radiology 2010;255(2):354–61.

19. Sprague BL, Arao RF, Miglioretti DL, et al. National performance benchmarks for modern diagnostic digital mammography: update from the Breast Cancer Surveillance Consortium. Radiology 2017; 283(1):59–69.

20. Ballard-Barbash R, Taplin SH, Yankaskas BC, et al. Breast Cancer Surveillance Consortium: a national mammography screening and outcomes database. AJR Am J Roentgenol 1997;169(4): 1001–8.

21. Pisano ED, Gatsonis C, Hendrick E, et al. Diagnostic performance of digital versus film mammography for breast-cancer screening. N Engl J Med 2005; 353(17):1773–83.

22. Patti JA. The national radiology data registry: a necessary component of quality health care. J Am Coll Radiol 2011;8(7):453.

23. Outcomes reported from the ACR National Mammography Database. Available at: https://nrdr.acr.org/Portal/NMD/Main/page.aspx. Accessed March 2, 2020.

24. D'Orsi CJ, Sickles EA. 2017 Breast Cancer Surveillance Consortium reports on interpretive performance at screening and diagnostic mammography: welcome new data, but not as benchmarks for practice. Radiology 2017;283(1):7–9.

25. Lee CS, Moy L, Friedewald SM, et al. Harmonizing breast cancer screening recommendations: metrics and accountability. AJR Am J Roentgenol 2018; 210(2):241–5.

26. Lee CS, Parise C, Burleson J, et al. Assessing the recall rate for screening mammography: comparing the Medicare hospital compare dataset with the National Mammography Database. AJR Am J Roentgenol 2018;211(1):127–32.

27. Nelson HD, Cantor A, Humphrey L, et al. Screening for breast cancer: a systematic review to update the 2009 U.S. Preventive Services Task Force Recommendation. Rockville (MD): Agency for Healthcare Research and Quality; 2016. January Report No.: 14-05201-EF-1.

28. Rothschild J, Lourenco AP, Mainiero MB. Screening mammography recall rate: does practice site matter? Radiology 2013;269(2):348–53.

29. Miglioretti DL, Ichikawa L, Smith RA, et al. Criteria for identifying radiologists with acceptable screening mammography interpretive performance on basis of multiple performance measures. AJR Am J Roentgenol 2015;204(4):W486–91.

30. Honig EL, Mullen LA, Amir T, et al. Factors impacting false positive recall in screening mammography. Acad Radiol 2019;26(11):1505–12.

31. Bitencourt AGV, Saccarelli CR, Morris EA. How to reduce false positive recall rates in screening mammography? Acad Radiol 2019;26(11):1513–4.

32. Rose SL, Tidwell AL, Ice MF, et al. A reader study comparing prospective tomosynthesis interpretations with retrospective readings of the corresponding FFDM examinations. Acad Radiol 2014;21(9): 1204–10.

33. Haas BM, Kalra V, Geisel J, et al. Comparison of tomosynthesis plus digital mammography and digital mammography alone for breast cancer screening. Radiology 2013;269(3):694–700.

34. Smith-Bindman R, Ballard-Barbash R, Miglioretti DL, et al. Comparing the performance of mammography screening in the USA and the UK. J Med Screen 2005;12(1):50–4.

35. Rosenberg RD, Seidenwurm D. Optimizing breast cancer screening programs: experience and structures. Radiology 2019;292(2):297–8.

36. Hoff SR, Myklebust TA, Lee CI, et al. Influence of mammography volume on radiologists' performance: results from breastscreen Norway. Radiology 2019;292(2):289–96.

37. Buist DS, Anderson ML, Haneuse SJ, et al. Influence of annual interpretive volume on screening mammography performance in the United States. Radiology 2011;259(1):72–84.

38. Smith-Bindman R, Chu P, Miglioretti DL, et al. Physician predictors of mammographic accuracy. J Natl Cancer Inst 2005;97(5):358–67.

39. Monticciolo DL, Newell MS, Hendrick RE, et al. Breast cancer screening for average-risk women: recommendations from the ACR Commission on breast imaging. J Am Coll Radiol 2017;14(9): 1137–43.

40. Oeffinger KC, Fontham ET, Etzioni R, et al. Breast cancer screening for women at average risk: 2015 guideline update from the American Cancer Society. JAMA 2015;314(15):1599–614.

Breast Magnetic Resonance Imaging Audit
Pitfalls, Challenges, and Future Considerations

Diana L. Lam, MD*, Janie M. Lee, MD, MSc

KEYWORDS

- Breast MRI Audit • MRI Benchmarks • MRI Outcome audit

KEY POINTS

- A medical outcomes audit is essential for assessing individual and facility-level interpretive performance.
- Rigorous use of the American College of Radiology (ACR) Breast Imaging Reporting and Data System (BI-RADS) terminology and assessments is critical to allow accurate data capture and coding, particularly in breast magnetic resonance (MR) imaging performed for extent of disease evaluation.
- Breast MR imaging audit data should be captured and reported similarly to the mammography audit, with separate data calculated for screening versus diagnostic indications.
- Current breast MR imaging auditing guidance does not address issues related to multimodality screening use, which can result in biased estimates of test performance. Revision of auditing methods to account for multimodality screening strategies are needed to improve performance estimates in medical outcomes audits.

BACKGROUND

The major goals of breast cancer screening are to find a high percentage of screen-detected cancers (cancer detection rate and sensitivity), which are more likely to be curable (minimal and early-stage, node-negative cancers), while decreasing harms such as morbidity and cost caused by additional imaging and tissue biopsies (abnormal interpretation rate and positive predictive value [PPV]).[1,2] A medical imaging outcomes audit allows for quality improvement through feedback to both individual radiologists and the entire practice compared with established benchmarks. In particular, the audit can ascertain whether individual radiologists are outside an acceptable range of performance in order to help the radiologists identify and target areas for improvement. Annual participation in the Mammography Quality

Standards Act (MQSA) medical audit also fulfills part 4, Practice Quality Improvement of the American Board of Radiology (ABR) Maintenance of Certification.[3]

The use of contrast-enhanced breast magnetic resonance (MR) imaging for early breast cancer detection has grown over the past few decades as several prospective studies showed increased sensitivity for detecting breast cancer in women with genetic or familial breast cancer predisposition.[4–10] In 2007, the American Cancer Society (ACS) published guidelines for breast MR imaging screening indications.[11] In 2010, the American College of Radiology (ACR) and Society of Breast Imaging published the breast MR imaging appropriateness criteria[12] and the ACR established a breast MR imaging accreditation program. Unlike the required audit for mammography, the United States Food and Drug Administration currently

Department of Radiology, University of Washington School of Medicine, 1144 Eastlake Avenue East, LG-200, Seattle, WA 98109, USA
* Corresponding author.
E-mail address: dllam@uw.edu

Radiol Clin N Am 59 (2021) 57–65
https://doi.org/10.1016/j.rcl.2020.09.002
0033-8389/21/© 2020 Elsevier Inc. All rights reserved.

does not have regulations that mandate a medical outcomes audit of a breast MR imaging practice. However, a breast MR imaging outcomes audit, which includes interpretation accuracy and appropriate clinical indication, is required for practice accreditation through the ACR breast MR imaging accreditation program.[13]

The most recent 2013 edition of the ACR Breast Imaging Reporting and Data System (BI-RADS) atlas aligned cross-modality BI-RADS terminology and created a follow-up and outcome and monitoring section focusing on the medical audit.[1] Breast MR imaging screening benchmarks were based on analysis of prospective screening MR imaging trials of women at high risk for breast cancer, because large-scale breast MR imaging performance data from the United States clinical practice had yet to be published. Since then, additional research has been performed to improve performance measures for both screening and diagnostic breast MR imaging.[9,14–22] This article provides a framework for performing a breast MR imaging audit in clinical practice incorporating ACR BI-RADS guidance and more recent data, clarifies common pitfalls, and discusses audit challenges related to evolving clinical practice.

OVERVIEW OF THE BREAST MAGNETIC RESONANCE IMAGING AUDIT

Similar to the more established mammography audit, the breast MR imaging audit involves gathering and analyzing data from several sources: the breast MR imaging report, subsequent imaging and biopsy recommendations, and breast biopsy and surgical pathology. To help with data analysis, a standardized reporting system for reporting and coding should be followed, and appropriate use of the ACR BI-RADS lexicon when interpreting breast MR imaging examinations is critical. It is also essential to have an organized system for correlation of biopsy results with positive MR imaging studies for outcomes tracking.

The MR imaging audit is based on the overall BI-RADS assessment at the examination level, according to the most actionable BI-RADS lesion category, with recommendations for core biopsy (BI-RADS category 4 or 5) superseding that of a biopsy-proven malignancy (BI-RADS category 6). Institutions may choose to report individual findings at the lesion level and/or breast level to facilitate coordination and communication of patient care. However, breast MR imaging studies with a BI-RADS category 6 assessment at the examination level

should not be included in the medical audit because this would skew certain performance parameters.

An audit should be calculated once every screening interval. In general, this is assumed to be every year, because this is the most common screening interval in the United States; however, if a facility uses a longer screening interval, such as 2 years, this length of time should be substituted. The audit should include data moving forward for at least 1 year to allow sufficient time for diagnostic procedures, pathology results, and outcomes data capture to produce meaningful audit outcomes.

DATA COLLECTION AND DEFINITIONS

The ACR BI-RADS atlas includes guidelines for data collection for both the basic clinically relevant audit and the more complete audit (**Box 1**).[1] A basic clinically relevant audit provides a minimum amount of data to assess interpretive performance. These data include the number of screening and diagnostic examinations performed over a period of time and ACR BI-RADS category 0, 3, 4, and 5 recommendations. Subsequent tissue diagnosis pathology results and minimal cancer staging information are also needed. Recommendations for performance metrics to be calculated for the basic clinically relevant audit for breast MR imaging are similar to those from a mammography audit and include cancer detection rate (CDR), sensitivity, specificity, positive predictive values for biopsy recommendation and for biopsies performed, as well as characteristics of cancers: median size of invasive cancers, percentages of minimal cancer, stage 0 or 1 cancers, and node-negative invasive cancers.

The ACR also encourages collecting additional data to perform a more complete audit, which can provide additional important performance information. This audit includes collecting data on history of prior breast MR imaging examinations (for prevalent vs incident performance metrics), patient breast cancer risk factors (indications for breast MR imaging), mammographic breast density, type of imaging findings, and whether or not the cancer was palpable at the time of imaging. The more complete audit also includes sensitivity and specificity performance calculations, for which linkage to a pathology database or regional cancer registry will be needed to capture these data. Facilities without linkage to these databases have difficulties capturing both true-positive and true-negative examinations for these calculations.[23]

Box 1
Data Collected - Basic Clinically Relevant Audit and More Complete Audit

1. **Modality or modalities.**

2. **Dates of audit period and total number of examinations in that period (usually a 12-month period).**

3. Risk factors:

   - Patient's age at the time of the examination.
   - Breast and ovarian cancer history: personal or family (especially premenopausal breast cancer in first-degree relative—mother, sister, or daughter).
   - Previous biopsy-proven hyperplasia with cellular atypia, or lobular carcinoma in situ (LCIS).
   - Hormone replacement therapy.
   - Breast density as estimated at mammography.

4. **Number and type of examination: screening** (asymptomatic), **diagnostic** (evaluation of clinical symptoms or signs suggesting the possibility of breast cancer, evaluation of screening-detected findings, short-interval follow-up examinations).[a]

5. First-time examination or not.

6. Number of recommendations for:

   - **Additional imaging evaluation (recall) (BI-RADS category 0 = "Need Additional Imaging Evaluation").**
   - Routine (usually annual) screening (BI-RADS category 1 = "Negative" and category 2 = "Benign").
   - **Short-interval follow-up (BI-RADS category 3 = "Probably Benign").**
   - **Tissue diagnosis (BI-RADS category 4 = "Suspicious" and category 5 = "Highly Suggestive of Malignancy").**

7. **Tissue diagnosis results: malignant or benign, for all ACR BI-RADS category 0, 3, 4 and 5 assessments (keep separate data for fine-needle aspiration, core biopsy and surgical biopsy cases). MQSA Final Rule requires that an attempt is made to collect tissue diagnosis results only for mammography examinations for which tissue diagnosis is recommended.**

8. Cancer data:

   - Imaging findings: mass, calcifications, other signs of malignancy (including architectural distortion and the several types of asymmetry), no signs of malignancy.
   - Palpable or nonpalpable at time of imaging examination
   - **Cancer staging: histologic type, invasive cancer size, nodal status, and tumor grade.**

9. **MQSA Final Rule also requires analysis of any known false-negative mammography examinations by attempting to obtain surgical and/or pathology results and by review of negative mammography examinations.**

Note: **Bolded** items indicate data included in the basic clinically relevant mammography audit.

[a] Separate audit statistics should be maintained for screening examinations and for each of the subtypes of diagnostic examinations.

From D'Orsi CJ, Sickles EA, Mendelson EB, et al. ACR BI-RADS® Atlas, Breast Imaging Reporting and Data System. Reston (VA): American College of Radiology; 2013; with permission.

Data Definitions

The following data definitions are defined by the ACR BI-RADS atlas.[1]

Screening examination: performed in asymptomatic women for early detection of clinically unsuspected breast cancer. For breast MR imaging, this includes surveillance examinations for asymptomatic women with a personal history of breast cancer and asymptomatic women with history of breast reconstruction.

Diagnostic examination: breast MR imaging performed for extent of disease for women with recent diagnosis of breast cancer before receipt of definitive treatment, patients with clinical signs or symptoms that may suggest breast cancer, problem solving (abnormal mammogram or ultrasonography examination), follow-up of a prior BI-RADS category 3 finding, or follow-up for neoadjuvant chemotherapy to assess for treatment response. Although the BI-RADS atlas indicates that diagnostic breast MR imaging may be performed for short-interval follow-up after breast conservation therapy, if the woman is asymptomatic, then classifying the MR imaging as a screening examination most closely aligns with the intent of the medical outcomes audit. Of additional note, examinations with BI-RADS category 6 assessments should not be included in the audit, because the purpose of the audit is to evaluate performance for breast cancer detection.

Positive examination: the images acquired for a breast MR imaging examination are the same regardless of whether the indication is screening or diagnostic. However, for auditing purposes, the positivity criterion varies with indication. For screening MR imaging examinations, BI-RADS category 0, 3, 4, or 5 results are considered positive, where additional evaluation with either imaging or tissue biopsy are recommended. The use of BI-RADS category 0 (additional imaging) on MR imaging should be an infrequent occurrence and used only if the images are technically inadequate or if there a different imaging modality is recommended to confirm a benign imaging findings (such as a lymph node on ultrasonography). For diagnostic MR imaging examinations, only BI-RADS category 4 or 5 results are considered positive where tissue diagnosis via biopsy is recommended.

Negative screening or diagnostic examination: this is when no tissue diagnosis is recommended. For screening MR imaging, only routine follow-up is recommended (BI-RADS category 1 or 2). For diagnostic MR imaging, BI-RADS category 1, 2, or 3 assessments are considered negative, because no tissue diagnosis is recommended. For BI-RADS category 3 assessments, when used for the first time on a screening breast MR imaging examination, the category 3 assessment is a positive screening result, because additional imaging is recommended; however, on subsequent short-interval follow-up diagnostic MR imaging, it would be coded as a negative diagnostic result given that a tissue diagnosis is not recommended.

Tissue diagnosis: this includes any pathologic diagnosis after an interventional procedure such as fine-needle aspiration, core needle biopsy, or excisional biopsy. A tissue diagnosis includes cases where a diagnostic aspiration was performed to differentiate between a complicated cyst versus a solid mass, even if the fluid obtained was not sent for cytologic analysis.

Cancer: a tissue diagnosis of breast cancer (ductal carcinoma in situ or invasive breast cancer) within the recommended screening interval after the imaging examination. Pathology diagnosis of high-risk lesions such as atypical ductal carcinoma, lobular neoplasia, or nonbreast cancers (sarcoma, lymphoma, metastasis to the breast)

Table 1
Breast magnetic resonance imaging screening benchmarks in American College of Radiology BI-RADS Atlas, Fifth Edition, compared with Breast Cancer Surveillance Consortium benchmarks

Benchmark	2013 BI-RADS Atlas, MR Imaging[a]	2017 BCSC Benchmarks
CDR (per 1000 examinations)	20–30	17
PPV2, recommendation for tissue diagnosis (%)	15	19
PPV3, biopsy performed (%)	20–50	21
False-positive biopsy recommendation rate (per 1000 examinations)	—	66
Sensitivity, if measurable (%)	>80	81
Specificity, if measurable (%)	85–90	83
Stage 0 or 1 cancer (%)	TBD	87
Node-negative invasive cancers (%)	>80	88
Median size of invasive cancers (mm)	TBD	10

Abbreviation: TBD, to be determined.
[a] Based on data from 5 prospective screening MR imaging trials of women with hereditary predisposition for breast cancer performed in Europe and Canada.[6,9,24–27]
Adapted from Lee JM, Ichikawa L, Valencia E, et al. Performance Benchmarks for Screening Breast MR Imaging in Community Practice. *Radiology.* 2017;285(1):44-52; with permission.

are not classified as true-positive or a cancer in the medical outcomes audit.

COMPARISON WITH BENCHMARKS

The medical outcomes audit is most useful for comparisons with standard benchmarks representative of the patient population. At the time of publication of the fifth edition of the ACR BI-RADS manual, the screening MR imaging benchmarks were based on prospective clinical trials of women at high risk of breast cancer, because there were insufficient breast MR imaging audit data from United States clinical practices.[6,9,24–28] Since 2013, additional studies have narrowed this knowledge gap.[14–17]

The largest screening breast MR imaging outcomes study used data from the National Cancer Institute–funded Breast Cancer Surveillance Consortium (BCSC), which includes a geographically and ethnically diverse sample of the United States population and breast imaging data from facilities linked to outcome data from state and regional tumor registries. This study found that most performance parameters met or approached the ACR BI-RADS benchmarks (Table 1), and also provided additional values for 2 benchmarks categorized as to be determined in the BI-RADS atlas: median size of invasive cancers and percentage of stage 0 or 1 cancer.[17] Multi-institutional diagnostic breast MR imaging outcomes data have yet to be published, although screening and diagnostic breast MR imaging examinations should be audited separately because there is significant difference in abnormal interpretation rates and other metrics based on clinical indication.[14,22]

Beyond the basic clinical audit for screening MR imaging, performance of the more complete audit is encouraged, to better understand the clinical practice. As more women receive screening breast MR imaging, the proportion of women with prior comparison breast MR imaging examinations increases, with studies showing improved interpretive performance with lower abnormal interpretation and false-positive biopsy rate during incidence breast MR imaging screening compared with prevalent baseline screening.[18,29,30] Recent single-institutional studies have shown differences in breast MR imaging performance depending on patient risk factors, with a higher CDR in patients with BRCA mutations compared with those with a family history of breast cancer[19] and a higher CDR and positive predictive value after biopsy (PPV3) for women with a personal history compared with family history of breast cancer.[16,20]

It is also important to understand the difference between benchmarks, which show existing interpretative performance, versus guidelines or acceptable ranges, which express desired performance that individuals or institutions should meet. In addition to considering performance by individual benchmark, performance at the individual or practice level should also include simultaneous consideration of multiple benchmarks, because the performance measures can be related. For example, a high abnormal interpretation rate associated with a high CDR would be considered appropriate for a clinical practice, because it suggests a higher-risk population being screened. However, a high abnormal interpretation rate associated with a low CDR suggests a high false-positive rate, which may be considered a screening harm.[31] Guidelines have been developed for screening mammography performance after critical review of data and expert opinion, but acceptable ranges of MR imaging performance have yet to be developed.[28]

COMMON PITFALLS AND CHALLENGES

Coding of Screening Versus Diagnostic Breast Magnetic Resonance Imaging Examinations

Although the definitions of screening versus diagnostic examination are clear based on indication, institutions may code certain examinations as a diagnostic examination for surveillance in women with personal history of breast cancer or in women with breast augmentation, even though the patient is asymptomatic. However, when conducting the medical outcomes audit, these examinations should be considered as screening examinations according to the ACR BI-RADS atlas.[28]

For surveillance mammography, observed variability in screening versus diagnostic coding across imaging facilities complicates assessment of mammography performance and outcomes. Within BCSC facilities, a substantial portion (39%) of mammography examinations in asymptomatic women with a personal history of breast cancer were coded as diagnostic examinations within the first 5 years of treatment completion, and particularly if women received breast conservation therapy.[32] For these women, audits of mammography performance that only include the screening indication systematically exclude an important subgroup and introduce bias into performance estimates. It is not yet clear whether surveillance MRI has similar variability for indication coding. This issue may be addressed by increased standardization of indication coding for asymptomatic women with treated breast cancer, perhaps with updated ACR guidance.

Incorrect Use of Breast Imaging Reporting and Data System Categories and Assessments

Accurate use of BI-RADS terminology and assessment categories in reporting is critical to an accurate audit. In the setting of the ACR's breast MR imaging interpretation course, radiologists were more likely to provide correct BI-RADS assessments on screening breast MR imaging examinations compared with diagnostic MR imaging examinations. A high percentage of incorrect responses was caused by categorizing suspicious masses and nonmass enhancement as BI-RADS category 6 instead of BI-RADS category 4 or 5. The highest number of incorrect BI-RADS assessments was observed in the setting of additional findings in a patient with recent biopsy-proven malignancy.[33]

For breast MR imaging examinations obtained to evaluate for extent of disease, if there are additional suspicious findings besides the known cancer that would change surgical management, such as an additional mass or nonmass enhancement that has yet to be biopsied, then a BI-RADS category 4 or 5 should be given to the lesion and the overall examination BI-RADS should be based on the most actionable finding using the BI-RADS hierarchy (5>4>0>6>3>2>1). Therefore, a recommendation of a biopsy (BI-RADS 4 or 5) supersedes a BI-RADS category 6 assessment, and the overall examination code for this diagnostic MR imaging should be a BI-RADS category 4 or 5, not a BI-RADS category 6.

Another common incorrect use of BI-RADS category 6 is in the postlumpectomy setting with positive margins, when MR imaging is requested to evaluate for residual disease. If there is no focal suspicious enhancement to suggest the presence of visible residual malignancy, the postsurgical changes should be given a BI-RADS category 2 assessment. If there are residual or additional suspicious findings on the breast MR imaging, then a BI-RADS category 4 or 5 should be rendered, not a BI-RADS category 6.

Multimodality Screening

As multimodality breast cancer screening for higher-risk women is increasingly used in clinical practice, challenges are created for auditing that are focused on independent assessment of each

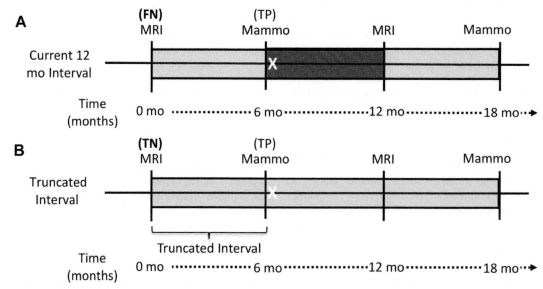

Fig. 1. Attribution of breast cancer with multimodality screening with overlapping follow-up periods. (A) Double counting of single cancer diagnosis: with an alternating screening strategy of screening MR imaging and mammography every 6 months, if the first screening MR imaging has a negative result and a cancer diagnosis (*white X*) is diagnosed after the subsequent screening mammogram with a positive result, this breast cancer will be double counted as a true-positive for the mammogram and false-negative for the MR imaging using current BI-RADS auditing guidance. Dark gray indicates overlapping screening interval. (B) Truncated follow-up: if the follow up interval is truncated at the time of the next screening examination, overlapping follow-up periods are eliminated. The breast cancer that was diagnosed would be counted only once and attributed to the screening mammogram that immediately preceded it (true-positive examination). The prior MR imaging examination would be classified as a true-negative examination. FN, false-negative; Mammo, mammogram; TP, true-positive.

breast imaging modality, whether mammography, ultrasonography, or MR imaging.

As an example, women at high risk for developing breast cancer are recommended to receive screening with both mammography and MR imaging to increase earlier breast cancer detection.[11,34,35] These examinations may be performed close together in time, usually within a month of each other,[21] or may be performed approximately 6 months apart.[36] Multimodality screening with alternating tests at intervals shorter than the standard follow-up period poses a particular auditing challenge, because it creates overlapping follow-up periods and complicates attribution of breast cancer outcomes. If the first screening examination has a negative result and a cancer is subsequently diagnosed after the second screening examination with a positive result, the breast cancer that is diagnosed may be double counted as both a true-positive for the second examination and a false-negative for the first examination (Fig. 1A). This finding was observed in the screening MR imaging study in community practice,[17] where 23% of interval cancers (8 of 35) diagnosed after negative breast MR imaging were subsequently detected with screening mammography performed within the 1-year follow-up period of the breast MR imaging examination. In addition, an additional 2 interval cancers (9%) were identified on screening MR imaging performed within 365 days of the prior MR imaging with negative results. In these cases, a single breast cancer was double counted as both true-positive for the subsequent test (either mammography or MR imaging) and a false-negative for the preceding MR imaging. This dual attribution of breast cancers that are screen detected on 1 examination and interval cancers associated with another screening modality artifactually reduces the sensitivity of the initial test in the sequence. Had these 10 false-negative cases been removed from the calculation of sensitivity in this study, breast MR imaging sensitivity would have increased from 81% to 85%.

Current BI-RADS auditing guidance does not address this issue of overlapping follow-up periods. As women increasingly pursue multimodality screening based on their breast cancer risk factors, revision of auditing methods to account for multimodality strategies in addition to single-modality assessments will be needed to improve medical outcomes audits. A possible solution to address this issue, especially when multimodality screening is performed at alternating 6-month intervals, might be to truncate the audit follow-up period of a screening test when an asymptomatic woman returns for her next screening test, regardless of modality (Fig. 1B). As an example, if a woman had breast MR imaging with a negative result and returned 6 months later for a screening mammogram, the follow-up period for the MR imaging examination would end on the date of the subsequent screening mammogram, and the outcome of the breast MR imaging examination would be classified as true-negative. If the screening mammogram had a positive result and a breast cancer was subsequently diagnosed, the breast cancer would only be attributed to the screening mammogram and classified as a true-positive. Truncating the audit follow-up period of the breast MR imaging removes the overlapping follow-up period for the alternating screening tests, even though they both occurred within a 1 year period. Elimination of the dual attribution of a single cancer as both true-positive for screening mammography and false-negative for MR imaging increases the calculated sensitivity of MR imaging.[37] By classifying the MR imaging in this example as a true-negative examination, the calculated specificity for MR imaging increases as well. As the BI-RADS atlas is updated for future editions, revised guidance for multimodality auditing would improve estimates of diagnostic performance and the impact of these strategies on outcomes.

SUMMARY

Breast MR imaging is the most sensitive imaging modality for breast cancer detection and guidelines recommend its use, in addition to screening mammography, for high-risk women with genetic and familial predisposition.[11,34,35] This recommendation has led to increased breast MR imaging use, including a large proportion of women with a personal history of breast cancer.[14,16,20] The most recent ACR BI-RADS manual coordinated cross-modality BI-RADS terminology, established an outcome and monitoring audit section, and published benchmarks for screening breast MR imaging primarily from research data at academic centers.[28] Since then, additional screening breast MR imaging benchmarks representative of United States community practice have been published; however, multi-institutional benchmarks and performance for diagnostic breast MR imaging are not yet available. Common pitfalls influencing audit results are discussed, and the effect of increasing multimodality screening use highlights areas of focus as auditing practices evolve.

ACKNOWLEDGMENTS

Dr J.M. Lee's contributions were supported in part by a grant from the National Cancer Institute, United States (P01CA154292).

DISCLOSURE

Dr J.M. Lee has a research grant from GE Healthcare, United States.

REFERENCES

1. D'Orsi CJ, Sickles EA, Mendelson EB, et al. ACR BI-RADS® Atlas, breast imaging reporting and data system. Reston (VA): American College of Radiology; 2013.
2. Tabar L, Fagerberg G, Duffy SW, et al. Update of the Swedish two-county program of mammographic screening for breast cancer. Radiol Clin North Am 1992;30(1):187–210.
3. Donnelly LF, Mathews VP, Laszakovits DJ, et al. Recent Changes to ABR Maintenance of Certification Part 4 (PQI): Acknowledgment of Radiologists' Activities to Improve Quality and Safety. J Am Coll Radiol 2016;13(2):184–7.
4. Stout NK, Nekhlyudov L, Li L, et al. Rapid increase in breast magnetic resonance imaging use: trends from 2000 to 2011. JAMA Intern Med 2014;174(1): 114–21.
5. Wernli KJ, DeMartini WB, Ichikawa L, et al. Patterns of breast magnetic resonance imaging use in community practice. JAMA Intern Med 2014;174(1): 125–32.
6. Kriege M, Brekelmans CT, Boetes C, et al. Efficacy of MRI and mammography for breast-cancer screening in women with a familial or genetic predisposition. N Engl J Med 2004;351(5):427–37.
7. Kuhl C, Weigel S, Schrading S, et al. Prospective multicenter cohort study to refine management recommendations for women at elevated familial risk of breast cancer: the EVA trial. J Clin Oncol 2010; 28(9):1450–7.
8. Lehman CD, Blume JD, Weatherall P, et al. Screening women at high risk for breast cancer with mammography and magnetic resonance imaging. Cancer 2005;103(9):1898–905.
9. Passaperuma K, Warner E, Causer PA, et al. Long-term results of screening with magnetic resonance imaging in women with BRCA mutations. Br J Cancer 2012;107(1):24–30.
10. Leach MO, Boggis CR, Dixon AK, et al. Screening with magnetic resonance imaging and mammography of a UK population at high familial risk of breast cancer: a prospective multicentre cohort study (MARIBS). Lancet 2005;365(9473):1769–78.
11. Saslow D, Boetes C, Burke W, et al. American Cancer Society guidelines for breast screening with MRI as an adjunct to mammography. CA Cancer J Clin 2007;57(2):75–89.
12. Lee CH, Dershaw DD, Kopans D, et al. Breast cancer screening with imaging: recommendations from the Society of Breast Imaging and the ACR on the use of mammography, breast MRI, breast ultrasound, and other technologies for the detection of clinically occult breast cancer. J Am Coll Radiol 2010;7(1):18–27.
13. American College of Radiology. Quality Assurance: Breast MRI. 2019. Available at: https://accreditation support.acr.org/support/solutions/articles/11000064333-quality-assurance-breast-mri-revised-12-12-19-. Accessed May 25, 2020.
14. Niell BL, Gavenonis SC, Motazedi T, et al. Auditing a breast MRI practice: performance measures for screening and diagnostic breast MRI. J Am Coll Radiol 2014;11(9):883–9.
15. Sedora Roman NI, Mehta TS, Sharpe RE, et al. Proposed biopsy performance benchmarks for MRI based on an audit of a large academic center. Breast J 2018;24(3):319–24.
16. Strigel RM, Rollenhagen J, Burnside ES, et al. Screening breast MRI outcomes in routine clinical practice: comparison to BI-RADS benchmarks. Acad Radiol 2017;24(4):411–7.
17. Lee JM, Ichikawa L, Valencia E, et al. Performance benchmarks for screening breast MR imaging in community practice. Radiology 2017;285(1):44–52.
18. Hayward JH, Ray KM, Price ER, et al. Performance of screening MRI in high risk patients at initial versus subsequent screen. Clin Imaging 2020;66:87–92.
19. Sippo DA, Burk KS, Mercaldo SF, et al. Performance of screening breast MRI across women with different elevated breast cancer risk indications. Radiology 2019;292(1):51–9.
20. Lehman CD, Lee JM, DeMartini WB, et al. Screening MRI in women with a personal history of breast cancer. J Natl Cancer Inst 2016;108(3):djv349.
21. Chiarelli AM, Blackmore KM, Muradali D, et al. Performance measures of magnetic resonance imaging plus mammography in the high risk ontario breast screening program. J Natl Cancer Inst 2020; 112(2):136–44.
22. Lee CI, Ichikawa L, Rochelle MC, et al. Breast MRI BI-RADS assessments and abnormal interpretation rates by clinical indication in US community practices. Acad Radiol 2014;21(11):1370–6.
23. Burnside ES, Woo K, Shafer C, et al. Current Recommended Methods for Calculating Screening Mammography Cancer Detection Rate Systematically Underestimate Performance Compared to Benchmarks. Abstract presented at 2017 Radiological Society of North America Annual meeting, Chicago, IL, November 27, 2017.
24. Warner E, Plewes DB, Hill KA, et al. Surveillance of BRCA1 and BRCA2 mutation carriers with magnetic resonance imaging, ultrasound, mammography, and clinical breast examination. JAMA 2004;292(11): 1317–25.
25. Leach MO, Brindle KM, Evelhoch JL, et al. The assessment of antiangiogenic and antivascular

therapies in early-stage clinical trials using magnetic resonance imaging: issues and recommendations. Br J Cancer 2005;92(9):1599–610.

26. Kuhl CK, Schrading S, Leutner CC, et al. Mammography, breast ultrasound, and magnetic resonance imaging for surveillance of women at high familial risk for breast cancer. J Clin Oncol 2005;23(33): 8469–76.

27. Sardanelli F, Podo F. Breast MR imaging in women at high-risk of breast cancer. Is something changing in early breast cancer detection? Eur Radiol 2007; 17(4):873–87.

28. Sickles EA, D'Orsi CJ. ACR BI-RADS® follow-up and outcome monitoring. In: D'Orsi CJ, editor. ACR BI-RADS® atlas, breast imaging reporting and data system. Reston (VA): American College of Radiology; 2013.

29. Burk KS, Edmonds CE, Mercaldo SF, et al. The Effect of Prior Comparison MRI on interpretive performance of screening breast MRI. J Breast Imaging 2020;2(1):36–42.

30. Vreemann S, Gubern-Mérida A, Schlooz-Vries MS, et al. Influence of risk category and screening round on the performance of an MR imaging and mammography screening program in carriers of the BRCA mutation and other women at increased risk. Radiology 2018;286(2):443–51.

31. Miglioretti DL, Ichikawa L, Smith RA, et al. Criteria for identifying radiologists with acceptable screening mammography interpretive performance on basis of multiple performance measures. AJR Am J Roentgenol 2015;204(4):W486–91.

32. Buist DSM, Ichikawa L, Wernli KJ, et al. Facility variability in examination indication among women with prior breast cancer: implications and the need for standardization. J Am Coll Radiol 2020;17(6): 755–64.

33. Lee CI, Grauke LJ, Sandhir V, et al. Radiologists' Performance in the ACR Breast MR With Guided Biopsy Course. J Am Coll Radiol 2013;10(11):854–8.

34. Monticciolo DL, Newell MS, Moy L, et al. Breast cancer screening in women at higher-than-average risk: recommendations from the ACR. J Am Coll Radiol 2018;15(3 Pt A):408–14.

35. National Comprehensive Cancer Network. Breast Cancer Screening and Diagnosis. Available at: www.NCCN.org. Accessed May 27, 2020, Version 1.2019.

36. Le-Petross HT, Whitman GJ, Atchley DP, et al. Effectiveness of alternating mammography and magnetic resonance imaging for screening women with deleterious BRCA mutations at high risk of breast cancer. Cancer 2011;117(17):3900–7.

37. Rosenberg RD, Yankaskas BC, Hunt WC, et al. Effect of variations in operational definitions on performance estimates for screening mammography. Acad Radiol 2000;7(12):1058–68.

Supplemental Screening for Patients at Intermediate and High Risk for Breast Cancer

Lilian Wang, MD[a,b], Roberta M. Strigel, MD, MS[c,*]

KEYWORDS

- Supplemental screening • High risk • Breast cancer • Intermediate risk

KEY POINTS

- Patients with an intermediate or high lifetime risk for breast cancer may benefit from supplemental screening beyond 2-dimensional mammography to improve the detection of breast cancer.
- Supplemental screening modalities beyond 2-dimensional mammography include digital breast tomosynthesis, contrast-enhanced spectral mammography, ultrasound examination, MR imaging, and molecular breast imaging.
- The decision to perform supplemental screening depends on individual risk status, evidence to support a specific modality for a given clinical scenario, cost, and availability.
- Prospective, multi-institutional trials of supplemental screening with direct comparison of the recall rate, cancer detection rate, and false-positive examinations are needed.

INTRODUCTION

The early detection of breast cancer with screening mammography in women who undergo screening has been well-established in multiple trials to decrease mortality by more than 40%.[1–7] However, the sensitivity of mammography is more limited in patients with dense breasts[8] and some patients at higher risk of breast cancer (as low as 19%–37%).[9–13] Patients with an intermediate or high lifetime risk for breast cancer may begin screening at an earlier age[14] and benefit from supplemental screening beyond standard 2-dimensional (2D) mammography to improve the early detection of breast cancer. The determination of whether or not supplemental screening is implemented for a given patient, and the modality chosen, is based on several factors. These parameters include the patient's individual risk factors for developing breast cancer (personal or family history of breast cancer, genetic mutation, history of atypia or lobular hyperplasia, nulliparity), imaging data such as mammographic breast density, and the evidence supporting a specific modality for supplemental screening given the clinical scenario. Additional factors for consideration include the availability of supplemental screening techniques at an individual institution, cost, insurance coverage, patient and physician preferences, and state-specific breast density legislation.

This article includes a review of risk profiles that may be considered for supplemental screening, breast density, types of supplemental screening modalities, and current national guidelines.

[a] Northwestern Medicine, Chicago, IL, USA; [b] Prentice Women's Hospital, 250 East Superior Street, 4th Floor, Room 04-2304, Chicago, IL 60611, USA; [c] Breast Imaging and Intervention, University of Wisconsin, 600 Highland Avenue, Madison, WI 53792-3252, USA
* Corresponding author.
E-mail address: RStrigel@uwhealth.org

Radiol Clin N Am 59 (2021) 67–83
https://doi.org/10.1016/j.rcl.2020.09.006
0033-8389/21/© 2020 Elsevier Inc. All rights reserved.

DISCUSSION
High-Risk Screening

Genetic predisposition

Hereditary breast and ovarian cancer syndrome reflects the presence of a genetic mutation that confers a higher risk for the development of breast and ovarian cancers. Inherited genetic mutations are implicated in approximately 5% to 10% of breast cancers, with the most common genetic mutations affecting the BRCA1 or BRCA2 genes.[15] The estimated lifetime risk for the development of breast cancer is up to 87% for a BRCA1 gene mutation carrier and 56% for a BRCA2 gene mutation carrier.[16] In patients with a known pathogenic (or likely pathogenic) BRCA gene mutation, screening is recommended to begin by age 25 (**Table 1**).[14,17–19]

Although BRCA1 and BRCA2 are the most well-known gene mutations, pathogenic variants in multiple other cancer predisposition genes may also increase risk for breast cancer.[20] Evidence characterizing breast cancer risk for certain gene mutations have led to additional recommendations for breast cancer screening in these patients,[20] including TP53 (Li–Fraumeni syndrome), CDH1 (hereditary gastric cancer syndrome), PALB2, ATM (ataxia–telangiectasia), NBN, CHEK2, STK11 (Peutz–Jeghers syndrome), and Cowden syndrome/PTEN hamartoma tumor syndrome.[18] The age at which to start and the modality of screening varies depending on the pathogenic variant (see **Table1**).

Family history

Patients without a known pathogenic variant in a gene conferring an increased risk for breast cancer, but with a significant family history of breast cancer, remain at higher risk for the development of breast cancer. Once a patient's lifetime risk reaches 20% or higher, supplemental screening with breast MR imaging in addition to mammography is recommended.[14,19,21] Individual risk assessment should be based on models that are largely dependent on family history, such as Claus, BRCAPRO, and Tyrer-Cuzick (IBIS).[14,19,21] Both the number of family members with breast cancer (particularly first-degree relatives) and their age at diagnosis are important considerations in addition to other factors depending on the specific model in use.[14] Screening begins between the ages of 25 and 30, or 10 years before the earliest affected relative (see **Table 1**).

Chest radiation

Women who have received radiation to fields encompassing the chest region that may include the breast tissue, such as thorax, whole lung, mediastinal, axilla, minimantle, subtotal lymphoid, high abdominal, and total body irradiation, are at higher risk for the development of breast cancer.[22,23] These women are most often survivors of childhood, adolescent, and young adult cancers such as Hodgkin's lymphoma and have much improved long-term survival compared with previous decades.[22] However, they are at substantially higher risk for the development of breast cancer, with a cumulative incidence of 13% to 20% by age 45, similar to that of BRCA gene mutation carriers.[22,24] Screening begins at age 25 or 8 to 10 years after the completion of radiation, whichever occurs last[14,22–24] (see **Table 1**).

Intermediate-Risk Screening

Personal history of breast cancer

Patients with a personal history of treated breast cancer are at higher risk for the development of a subsequent breast cancer. This second breast cancer could be a second primary tumor in either breast or a recurrence in the breast, chest wall, or axillary or internal mammary lymph nodes. After undergoing breast conservation therapy, the recurrence rate is 0.5% to 1.0% per year and the risk to develop a second cancer is 5% to 10% in the first decade after diagnosis[25]; and survival is known to improve with the early detection of a second breast cancer.[26] Screening mammography has a lower sensitivity in patients with a personal history of treated breast cancer.[27] Thus, some guidelines[14] support the use of supplemental screening in this patient population, particularly in those patients with dense breasts or a younger age at diagnosis (<50 year old).[14]

High-risk lesions

A personal history of biopsy proven lobular neoplasia (lobular carcinoma in situ or atypical lobular hyperplasia) or atypical ductal hyperplasia (ADH) increases risk for the subsequent development of breast cancer. The increased risk is most significant with lobular neoplasia, which portends a lifetime risk of 10% to 20%.[28] ADH also increases risk, but to a lesser degree than lobular carcinoma in situ. The relative risk for invasive cancer owing to ADH is 4- to 5-fold higher, but it is 6- to 10-fold higher for lobular carcinoma in situ.[14,29] Imaging surveillance typically begins at diagnosis (see **Table 1**).

Dense breasts

Mammographic breast density is routinely categorized into 1 of 4 categories by the interpreting radiologist during clinical mammographic interpretation.[30,31] Approximately 50% of women are in the 2 highest breast density categories

Table 1
ACR and NCCN guidelines for breast cancer screening by risk category

Patient Group	ACR	NCCN
BRCA[14,18]	MR imaging ≥25–30 y MG ≥30 y[b]	MR imaging ≥25–29 y to 75 y[a] MG ≥30–75 y
Li–Fraumeni syndrome (TP53)[14,18]	MR imaging ≥25–30 y MG ≥30 y	MR imaging ≥20–29 y to 75 y MG ≥30–75 y >75: Individual management
Cowden syndrome/PTEN hamartoma tumor syndrome[14,18]	MR imaging ≥25–30 y MG ≥30 y	MG + MR imaging 30–35 y[c] to 75 y
Peutz-Jeghers syndrome (STK11)[14,113]	MR imaging ≥25–30 y MG ≥30 y	MG + MR imaging ≥25y
CHEK2/ATM/NBN with 657del5 variant[14,18]	MR imaging ≥25–30 y MG ≥30 y	MG + consider MR imaging ≥40 y
PALB2/CDH1[14,18]	MR imaging ≥25–30 y MG ≥30 y	MG + MR imaging ≥30y
NF1[18]	Not specifically discussed	MG ≥30 y Consider MR imaging 30–50y
Untested first-degree relatives of mutation carriers[14,21]	MR imaging ≥25–30 y MG ≥30 y	Recommend
≥20% lifetime risk owing to family history[14,21]	MG ≥30 y MR imaging ≥25–30 y	MG + MR imaging 10y before youngest family member MR imaging not <25 y[d] MG not <30 y[d]
Chest radiation[14,21]	MG + MR imaging age 25 or 8 y after treatment[d]	MG + MR imaging 10 y after treatment No MG <30 y[d]
LCIS or ADH/ALH[14,21]	MG begin at diagnosis Consider MR imaging No MG <30 y[e] No MR imaging <25 y[e]	MG begin at diagnosis Consider MR imaging
Dense breasts (alone)[14,21]	MG ≥40 y Consider US ≥40 y MR imaging: Insufficient data MBI: not recommended	MG ≥40 y MR imaging: Insufficient evidence US: Can increase CDR, but may increase recall/benign biopsies MBI: Not recommended
Personal history of treated breast cancer[14,110]	MG begin at diagnosis MR imaging recommended if dense breasts or diagnosis <50 y[e]	Consider MR imaging if lifetime risk of second primary cancer >20%

Abbreviations: ACR, American College of Radiology; ADH, atypical ductal hyperplasia; ALH, atypical lobular hyperplasia; LCIS, lobular carcinoma in situ; MG, mammography with or without DBT; NCCN, National Comprehensive Cancer Network; US, ultrasound.
[a] Individualize for >75 y and family history <30 y.
[b] BRCA1 may consider delaying MG until 40.
[c] Or 5–10 y before the earliest breast cancer, whichever first.
[d] Whichever is later.
[e] Consider in all others.

(heterogeneously and extremely dense) (**Fig. 1**).[30] Compared with women of average breast density (between categories b and c), the relative risk of developing breast cancer if the breasts are heterogeneously dense is less than 1.2 and for extremely dense breasts it is less than 2.1.[32–38] Dense breasts increase the risk for the development of breast cancer, and patients in the highest

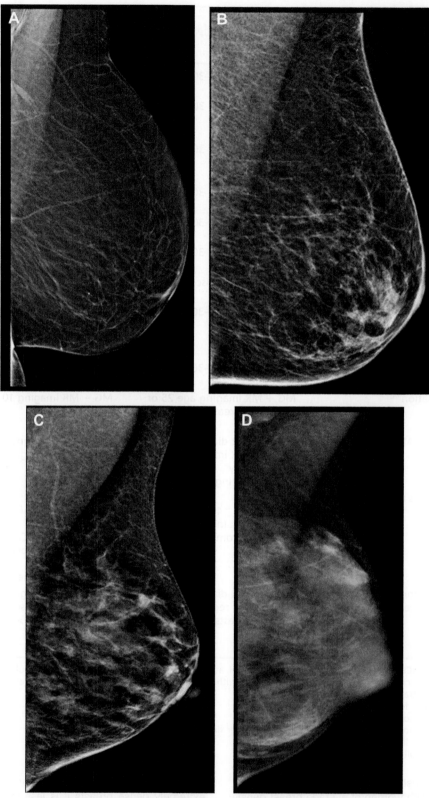

Fig. 1. Breast density categories depicted on representative mediolateral oblique mammographic views. (*A*) Almost entirely fatty (10% of patients). (*B*) Scattered areas of fibroglandular density (40% of patients). (*C*) Heterogeneously dense (40% of patients). (*D*) Extremely dense (10% of patients).

density category (extremely dense) have a 4 to 6 times greater likelihood of developing breast cancer than those in the lowest breast density category (fatty), although caution should be taken with this sort of comparison because less than 10% of the population fall into either of those 2 extreme categories.[39,40] Dense breasts also have a well-known masking effect on mammography, decreasing the sensitivity for breast cancer detection.[33] Some studies support supplemental screening beyond 2D mammography in patients with dense breasts given the combination of decreased mammographic sensitivity and increased risk for breast cancer.[41]

After legislation at a state-by-state level, federal breast density notification requirements were passed in 2019. These requirements direct the US Food and Drug Administration to implement breast density reporting requirements via the Mammography Quality Standard Act. Once implemented, the federal guidelines will require that mammography reports and summaries received by patients and their providers include information about the effect of breast density in masking the presence of breast cancer on a mammogram, the qualitative density assessment given by the radiologist who interpreted the mammogram, and a reminder to patients that they should talk with their provider if they have dense breasts and have questions or concerns. Some state-specific legislation also mentions supplemental screening and may legislate insurance coverage, although insurance coverage inclusion is less common.[42]

Modalities

Digital breast tomosynthesis

Digital breast tomosynthesis (DBT) is a digital mammogram technique in which tomosynthesis images are constructed from multiple low-dose images acquired as the x-ray source moves in an arc over the breast.[43] Compared with standard digital mammography (DM), DBT decreases the masking effect by decreasing superimposition from overlying breast parenchyma.[44] Both prospective and retrospective studies have demonstrated decreased recall rates and increased cancer detection rates (CDRs) with DBT compared with DM alone (**Fig. 2**).[45–47]

Although screening outcomes for DBT in specific high-risk populations are limited, because most studies did not include patient-level risk factors, the effects of DBT in higher risk women are likely similar to those described in average risk women. A retrospective study including 2673 women at increased risk (owing to personal history or first degree relative with breast cancer) reported a higher CDR for combined DBT and DM versus DM alone in both women at average risk (5.1 vs 4.5 per 1000) and increased risk (8.6 vs 7.9 per 1000); however, this difference was not statistically significant.[48] In a prospective study of 618 women with a personal history of breast cancer, the addition of DBT decreased the recall rate when compared with DM alone.[49] In contrast, in a randomized trial of women in their forties with a family history of breast cancer, the addition of DBT to DM in incident screening did not lead to a significant reduction in recall rate, although the DM recall rate was very low at 2.8%.[50] Data from the Tomosynthesis Mammographic Imaging Screening Trial (TMIST), which will include patient age, cancer risk, and breast density, will hopefully provide more information on screening outcomes for DBT in high-risk populations.[51]

For intermediate-risk women with dense breasts, DBT screening has a pooled incremental CDR (ICDR) beyond standard 2D mammography of 3.9 per 1000 in prospective screening trials and of 1.4 per 1000 in retrospective studies, with a significant decrease in the recall rate, with a pooled difference of −23.3 recalls per 1000 screens.[52] Overall, DBT screening in women with dense breasts is estimated to have an ICDR of 1 to 3 per 1000 examinations, a positive predictive value of biopsy (PPV3) of 25%, and a recall rate of 7% to 11%.[53,54]

Although studies have demonstrated improved CDRs and a decrease in the recall rates with DBT across breast density categories, including in women with dense breasts, cancers can be obscured if there is lack of a visible interface between the lesion and surrounding breast parenchyma. This factor may account for the higher ICDR seen with supplemental screening ultrasound (7.1 per 1000) compared with supplemental DBT (4 per 1000) in women with dense breasts and negative DM in the ASTOUND trial,[55] although at the expense of a significantly increased false-positive rate for ultrasound examinations.[56] Given that DBT detected more than 50% of additional breast cancers compared with DM alone, however, it is likely a superior primary screening modality for women with dense breasts compared with conventional 2D DM,[55] and may be considered for primary screening per National Comprehensive Cancer Network[21] and American College of Radiology[57] guidelines.

Contrast-enhanced spectral mammography

Contrast-enhanced spectral mammography (CESM) is an emerging technique that combines morphologic data from DM with functional data

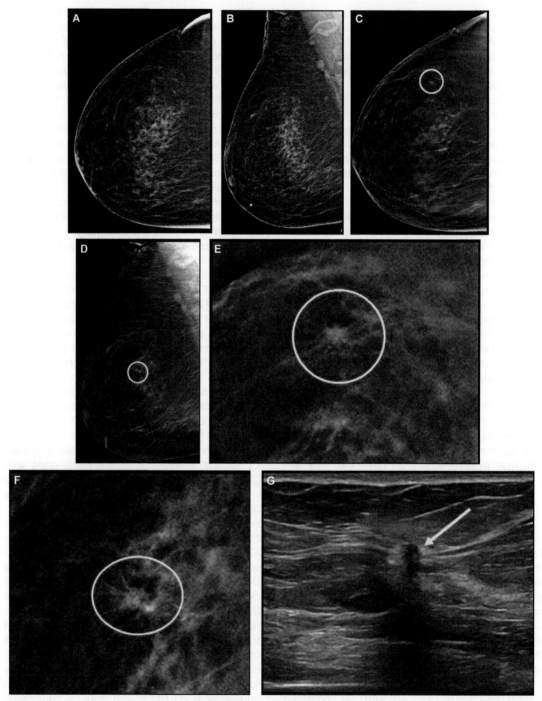

Fig. 2. A 61-year-old woman with a personal history of treated left breast cancer. Craniocaudal (CC) (*A*) and medial lateral oblique (MLO) (*B*) 2D full-field DM views from screening mammography demonstrate heterogeneously dense breasts and are otherwise negative. CC DBT (*C, E*) and MLO DBT (*D, F*) views demonstrate a 5-mm irregular, spiculated mass (*yellow circles*). (*G*) Targeted ultrasound image demonstrates a corresponding 5-mm irregular, hypoechoic, antiparallel mass with spiculated margins and posterior acoustic shadowing (*yellow arrow*). Biopsy demonstrated invasive ductal carcinoma.

from iodinated contrast uptake secondary to tumor angiogenesis for breast cancer detection.[58]

A meta-analysis of CESM reported a pooled sensitivity of 98% and specificity of 58%.[59] In a study of 72 women with dense breasts who underwent CESM and mammography, CESM had significantly higher accuracy (90.9%), sensitivity (86.2%), and specificity (94.1%) compared with mammography.[60] Although most studies have focused on the diagnostic usefulness of CESM, few studies have investigated its use as a screening tool. A pilot study comparing screening CESM and MR imaging for women at increased risk for breast cancer found that both modalities identified cancers not seen on DM, with a CESM recall rate of 7.5%, a PPV3 of 15.4%, and a specificity of 94.7%.[61] In a study of 611 women at intermediate risk who have dense breasts, screening CESM was significantly more sensitive than DM (90.5% vs 52.4%), with a specificity of 76.1%; a PPV of 11.9%; a negative predictive value of 99.6%; and an ICDR of 13.1 per 1000. Seven of 8 cancers seen only with CESM were invasive (mean size, 9 mm).[62] Results of a larger study of 904 women at increased risk undergoing screening CESM reported improved performance compared with DM, with increase in sensitivity from 50.0% to 87.5%; a specificity of 93.7%; a PPV3 of 29.4%; an ICDR of 6.6 per 1000; and a BI-RADS category 3 rate of 2.8%.[63]

Whole breast ultrasound examination

Ultrasound examination has several unique benefits as a supplemental screening modality: it is widely available, relatively inexpensive, well-tolerated by patients, and does not involve intravenous contrast administration (as with MR imaging) or radiation (as with molecular breast imaging [MBI]). Screening breast ultrasound examinations may be performed via handheld technique (technologist or physician) or automated scanner, and interpreted in either real time or batch fashion akin to screening mammography.

Multiple studies have demonstrated the usefulness of screening breast ultrasound imaging in identifying mammographically occult cancers, with an ICDR of 1.8 to 4.6 per 1000 women screened (**Fig. 3**).[64] Of incremental cancers identified via screening breast ultrasound, the majority are small (mean size, 10 mm), invasive, node-negative cancers.[64] By detecting cancers masked by breast parenchyma on mammography, supplemental screening ultrasound examination decreased the interval cancer rate by 50% in the Japan Strategic Anti-Cancer Randomized Trial (J-START).[65] A study of women with breast cancers detected at screening ultrasound

examination reported excellent outcomes, with a 5-year overall survival rate of 100% and recurrence-free survival rate of 98%.[66]

In high-risk women undergoing both screening mammography and MR imaging, ultrasound examination does not yield any additional cancer detection and should be reserved for further evaluation or biopsy of abnormalities identified on mammography or MR imaging.[11,67-69] For women with an increased risk who qualify for but cannot undergo MR imaging (for reasons including implants or devices incompatible with MR imaging, severe claustrophobia, and body habitus), supplemental screening with ultrasound examination should be considered.[14] The American College of Radiology Imaging Network 6666 trial was a multicenter prospective trial evaluating the performance of physician handheld screening ultrasound examinations in women with an increased risk and dense breast parenchyma. The ICDR for ultrasound examination was 5.3 per 1000 during the prevalence round and 3.7 per 1000 during the 2 incidence rounds, for an average ICDR of 4.3 per 1000.[70,71] This increased cancer detection, however, was offset by increased false positives, with a false-positive rate of ultrasound examination alone of 8.1% (vs 4.4% for mammography). The PPV3 for ultrasound-only findings was 9% for prevalence screening and 11.7% for incidence screening (vs 38.1% for mammography). Although performance improved with increased experience and comparison examinations, there was still a substantial rate of biopsy secondary to ultrasound screening, averaging 5% of all participants. After 3 rounds of screening with mammography and ultrasound examination, a subset of patients also underwent screening MR imaging, with an ICDR of 14.7 per 1000, demonstrating that ultrasound examination may still miss many cancers detected by MR imaging.

After the implementation of breast density legislation in Connecticut, data for technician-performed handheld ultrasound in women in the general population with dense breast parenchyma was published, with ICDR of 3.2 per 1000 and a PPV3 of 6.5% to 6.7%, lower than values reported for patients at elevated risk.[72,73] In women with dense breasts undergoing screening ultrasound examination, a retrospective study found no significant difference in additional cancer detection after DM versus after DBT.[74]

Factors limiting the implementation of screening breast ultrasound examinations include operator dependence,[64,75] a high-false positive rate (with recall rates twice as high and biopsy rates 2-3 times as high as screening mammography),[76] a low PPV of biopsy recommendations,[71,72] and a

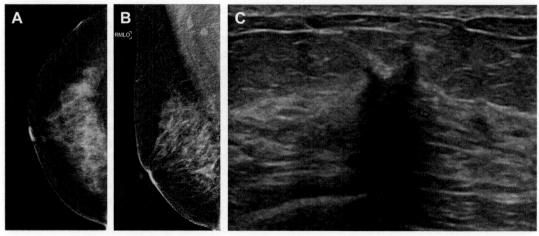

Fig. 3. A 55-year-old woman with dense breast parenchyma undergoing handheld technologist-performed screening ultrasound examination. Right craniocaudal (*A*) and medial lateral oblique (*B*) 2D full-field DM views from 2D-DBT screening mammography demonstrate heterogeneously dense breasts but are otherwise negative. (*C*) Ultrasound image demonstrates a 17-mm irregular hypoechoic mass with spiculated margins and antiparallel orientation at 12:00. Biopsy demonstrated grade 1 invasive lobular carcinoma.

high rate of BI-RADS 3 lesions requiring short-interval follow-up, ranging from 9% to 20%,[71–73] The technique is also time and labor intensive, with mean performance times ranging from 4 to 19 minutes for physician handheld ultrasound examination[70,77] and 10 minutes for technologist handheld ultrasound examination.[78]

Owing to the known limitations of handheld ultrasound examination, automated breast ultrasound (ABUS) examination systems have been developed to eliminate physician time for image acquisition and minimize operator dependence (**Fig. 4**). Studies have shown improved performance with the combination of mammography and ABUS examination.[79–81] Kelly and colleagues[79] showed an ICDR of 3.6 per 1000 screening examinations in women with dense breasts at increased risk for breast cancer undergoing ABUS examination. In a multi-institutional study evaluating more than 15,000 asymptomatic women with dense breasts, ABUS examination detected an additional 1.9 cancers per 1000 women.[80] Another study of ABUS examination in women with dense breasts reported an ICDR of 2.4 per 1000 with 9 additional recalls per 1000 women screened.[81]

The disadvantages of ABUS examination include shadowing from noncontact or Cooper's ligaments, limited visualization or coverage of peripheral lesions, shadowing behind the nipple, limited imaging with large breast size, and an inability to image the axillae. There may also be increased time and costs associated with need for recall and increased interpretation time given the number of images generated. Reported ABUS interpretation times range from 2.9 to 10.0 minutes,[79–81] longer than that for screening mammography but shorter than that for performance of physician handheld ultrasound examination.

In a comparative modeling study, the addition of ultrasound examination for women with dense breasts aged 50 to 74 averted an estimated 0.36 additional breast cancer deaths but resulted in 354 unnecessary benign biopsies per 1000 women screened.[82] Given high rates of recall and false-positive biopsy, the authors concluded that screening ultrasound examination is likely not cost effective and may cause greater harm than benefit.[82]

Breast MR imaging

Breast MR imaging is the most sensitive modality for the detection of breast cancer.[83] Multiple studies performed in the early 2000s studied the use of mammography and breast MR imaging for screening patients at high lifetime risk to develop breast cancer.[11,67–69,84–86] These patients were typically genetic mutation carriers or had a greater than 20% lifetime risk of developing breast cancer given a strong family history. In these trials, the sensitivity of mammography was 37%, the sensitivity of MR imaging was 82%, and the sensitivity of both mammography and MR imaging was the highest at 91%.[11,67–69,84–86] The additional supplemental yield of MR imaging beyond mammography was 28 cancers per 1000 examinations with a PPV3 (for biopsy) of 20% to 50% or higher.

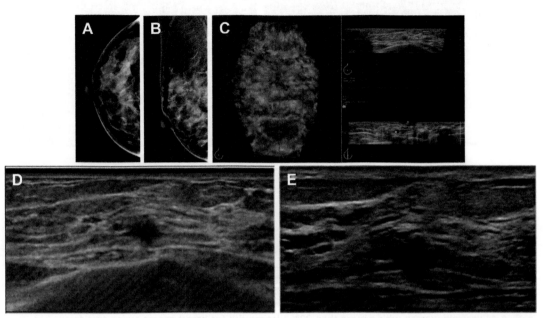

Fig. 4. A 44-year-old woman with dense parenchyma undergoing screening ABUS examination. Right craniocaudal (*A*) and medial lateral oblique (*B*) 2D full-field DM views from 2D-DBT screening mammography demonstrate heterogeneously dense breasts but are otherwise negative. (*C*) View from ABUS workstation demonstrating an 8-mm irregular hypoechoic subareolar breast mass in coronal, transverse, and sagittal planes, as visualized on (*D*) ABUS acquisition and (*E*) subsequent handheld ultrasound images. Biopsy revealed invasive lobular carcinoma.

Women at high risk for breast cancer owing to radiation to the chest also benefit from MR imaging screening. The sensitivity of mammography in these patients is 69% (range, 60%–72%) and the sensitivity of MR imaging is 76% (range, 67%–92%).[87–90] Compared with women with a hereditary predisposition for breast cancer, the sensitivity of MR imaging is lower and that of mammography higher.[24] The highest sensitivity (close to 95%) is achieved using both mammography and MR imaging in combination.[24]

For women at intermediate risk for the development of breast cancer, MR imaging may also have a role. Multiple studies of patients with a personal history of treated breast cancer have now demonstrated a CDR of 10 to 29 cancers per 1000 in this population.[91–98] In some studies, breast MR imaging performance is improved in patients with a personal history of breast cancer compared with those with a genetic or familial predisposition, with fewer false positives and higher specificity, CDR, and PPV3 (for biopsy).[94,96] Women at an increased risk owing to a personal history of lobular neoplasia or ADH may also benefit from supplemental screening with MR imaging,[99,100] particularly if they have an elevated risk of more than 20% or dense breasts (**Fig. 5**).[14,21]

The performance of MR imaging is not limited by increased breast density, and multiple studies

have evaluated the performance of breast MR imaging in women with dense breasts. The multicenter, randomized, controlled DENSE Trial evaluated women with extremely dense breasts between the ages of 50 and 75 years.[101] Women either received mammography screening only or were invited to also undergo supplemental screening MR imaging. The interval cancer rate was twice as high in the mammography-only group (5.0 per 1000 screens) versus the MR imaging invitation group (2.5 per 1000 screenings). For those women who actually underwent MR imaging, the CDR was 16.5 per 1000 screenings. The multicenter Eastern Cooperative Oncology Group–American College of Radiology Imaging Network 1141 trial recruited 1516 women aged 40 to 75 years with dense breasts (heterogeneously or extremely dense) undergoing routine mammographic screening with DBT to undergo supplemental abbreviated MR imaging screening.[102] The CDR was 11.8 per 1000 women for abbreviated breast MR imaging versus 4.8 per 1000 women for DBT (*P* = .002), demonstrating the potential benefit of even a limited MR imaging in this patient population (**Fig. 6**).[102]

Molecular breast imaging

MBI is a functional imaging technique that uses dedicated gamma cameras to image the

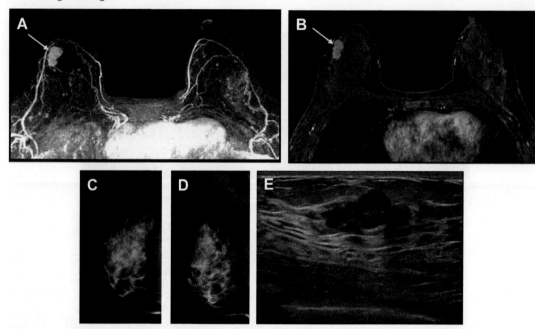

Fig. 5. A 44-year-old woman with a more than 20% lifetime risk for breast cancer owing to a family history of breast cancer and personal history of lobular carcinoma in situ. (*A*) The 3D maximum intensity projection axial T1-weighted early phase postcontrast subtraction MR images demonstrate a mass in the right breast (*yellow arrow*). (*B*) Axial T1-weighted early phase postcontrast MR images demonstrate a 20-mm irregular mass with circumscribed margins and homogeneous internal enhancement (BI-RADS category 4, suspicious). (*C*) Craniocaudal and (*D*) medial lateral oblique 2D mammographic views demonstrate heterogeneously dense breasts and are otherwise negative. (*E*) Targeted ultrasound examination after MR imaging demonstrates a 20-mm irregular, hypoechoic mass with indistinct margins which correlates with the MR imaging finding (biopsy result showed invasive ductal carcinoma).

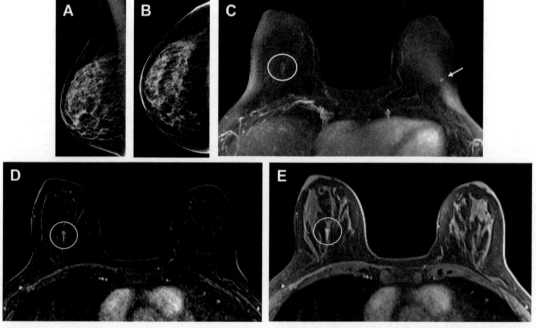

Fig. 6. A 71-year-old woman with dense breast parenchyma undergoing abbreviated breast MR imaging. Right (*A*) medial lateral oblique and (*B*) craniocaudal views demonstrate heterogeneously dense breast parenchyma. An area of non-mass enhancement is seen in the central right breast (*yellow circle*) on (*C*) maximum intensity projection (MIP), (*D*) axial postcontrast subtraction, and (*E*) axial postcontrast nonsubtraction MR images. MR imaging biopsy revealed DCIS. The enhancing mass in the outer left breast (*white arrow*) on (*C*) MIP image was mammographically stable and considered benign.

physiologic uptake of ^{99m}Tc-sestamibi within the breast tissue. Breast-specific gamma imaging (BSGI) uses a sodium iodide detector, whereas MBI uses dual-head cadmium zinc telluride detectors, with both systems collectively referred to as MBI. MBI is not limited by breast density and relies in part on tumor neovascularity to identify potential cancers.[103] A meta-analysis of BSGI as an adjunct to mammography showed a pooled sensitivity of 95% and specificity of 80%,[104] whereas 2 prospective single-center trials of MBI showed a combined sensitivity of 81.5% and specificity of 93.0%.[105,106]

In a study of supplemental screening BSGI in women at increased risk (mostly secondary to family and personal history of breast cancer), BSGI was reported to have an ICDR of 16.5 cancers per 1000 women screened.[107] In this series, the majority of cancers detected by BSGI were DCIS (57%). Studies evaluating MBI for screening women with dense breasts have described an ICDR ranging from 7.5 to 8.8 per 1000, with median cancer size of 1.0 cm, a recall rate of 5.9% to 8.4%, and a PPV3 of 19% to 33%.[103,105,106] In a study of 936 women with dense breasts, the sensitivity for breast cancer detection increased from 27% for mammography alone to 91% with combination of mammography and MBI, with similar specificity for MBI (93%) and mammography (91%).[106] Of cancers detected only by screening MBI, the majority were invasive (76%), with 24% demonstrating invasive lobular histology.

A limitation of MBI for screening is the associated radiation risk, which includes whole body radiation exposure. Initial studies using MBI used 20 to 30 mCi (740–1100 MBq) of ^{99m}Tc sestamibi.[108]

Recent studies have reported doses of 5 to 10 mCi[108]; the effective dose from MBI performed with 300 MBq (8 mCi) of ^{99m}Tc-sestamibi is approximately 2.4 mSv, compared with 0.5 to 1.2 mSv for mammography and DBT.[103] Recent advances in technology show promise in reducing radiation dose.[109] Regardless, MBI exposes all organs of the body to ionizing radiation and thus poses a higher risk of radiation-caused cancer and cancer deaths.[17]

Summary

A comparison between the different supplemental screening modalities for patients with dense breasts is included in **Table 2**. A summary of the benefits and drawbacks of all supplemental screening modalities is detailed in **Table 3**.

Supplemental Screening Guidelines

All major guidelines support the use of mammography, with or without DBT, to screen patients at increased risk for breast cancer, including the American College of Radiology,[14] National Comprehensive Cancer Network,[18,21,110] and the American Cancer Society.[19] Screening breast MR imaging is supported for supplemental screening in patients at high risk for breast cancer and in some patients at intermediate risk. Ultrasound examination is considered in the high-risk scenario if the patient cannot undergo MR imaging. Currently, the only guidelines to support possible consideration of supplemental screening with ultrasound examination in women with an elevated risk limited to increased breast density are the American College of Radiology guidelines (after weighing benefits and risks).[14,111] MBI and

Table 2
Comparison of supplemental screening modalities for dense breasts

Modality	Additional Time to Perform (min)	ICDR/1000	Radiation Dose			IV Injection
			Breast (mGy)	Body (mSv)	PPV3 (%)	
Ultrasound examination[48,58,64,72]	4–19	1.8–4.6	0	0	6–8	None
DBT (2 views)[17,46,48]	0	1.4–3.9	3.0–4.5	0.4–0.5	25	None
Breast MR imaging[65,96]	30	14.7–16.5	0	0	23–26	GBCA
Abbreviated breast MR imaging[97]	10	9.0	0	0	20	GBCA
MBI[98,100,101]	40	7.5–8.8	0.5	2.0–2.5	19–33	99mTc-sestamibi
CESM (2 views)[17,52,56,57]	8	6.6–13.1	3.6–4.5	0.4–0.5	24–29	Iodinated contrast

Abbreviations: GBCA, gadolinium based contrast agent; ICDR, incremental cancer detection rate; mGy, milliGray; mSv, milliSievert.

Table 3
Benefits and drawbacks of supplemental screening modalities

Modality	Benefits	Drawbacks
Ultrasound examination	Widely available, no ionizing radiation, not subject to breast density, well-tolerated by patients, less expensive than MR imaging	Operator dependent, time intensive, increased false positives, low positive predictive value, high rate of BI-RADS 3, limited chest wall visualization and coverage of large breasts with ABUS
DBT	Uses existing mammography equipment, no additional radiation dose beyond DM if using synthesized mammography	Increased radiation dose compared with DM alone if done in combination mode (DM + DBT), longer interpretation times, increased data storage requirement
Breast MR imaging	No ionizing radiation, highest sensitivity for breast cancer detection, high negative predictive value, functional examination with preferential detection of biologically aggressive cancers, BPE as potential marker for breast cancer risk, chest wall/axillary visualization	Requires IV, gadolinium deposition, time intensive, more expensive, not as widely available as mammography and ultrasound, may be less tolerable in patients with claustrophobia, may be contraindicated in those with pacemakers, metallic foreign bodies, impaired renal function, increased body mass index
Abbreviated breast MR imaging	Same as above, but less expensive and faster to perform and interpret than standard breast MR imaging	Same as above
MBI	Functional examination, claustrophobia-free apparatus, absence of renal toxicity, shorter interpretation time than DBT, ABUS, and MR imaging	Not widely available, requires IV injection of radiotracer, whole body radiation dose, longer examination time, validation needed for commercially available dual-headed biopsy system, lack of chest wall/axillary visualization
CESM	Functional examination, implemented using modification of existing mammography equipment, performed at time of standard mammogram, shorter imaging and interpretation time compared with MR imaging, no claustrophobia	Increased radiation dose compared with DM, requires IV iodinated contrast, risk of contrast-induced nephropathy, potential contrast reaction (severe acute reaction rate 0.04% vs 0.001%–0.01% for GBCA),[114] lack of chest wall/axillary visualization, lack of commercially available system for biopsy

Abbreviations: BPE, background parenchymal enhancement; GBCA, gadolinium-based contrast agent.

CESM are not endorsed for screening by any major organization at this time (see **Table 1**).

SUMMARY

There is currently much interest in the appropriate clinical scenarios and the best imaging modalities beyond mammography for supplemental screening for breast cancer. Determination of the best supplemental screening tool for a given clinical scenario will likely require prospective, multi-institutional trials with direct comparison of the recall rate, CDR, and false-positive examinations, balanced with additional considerations such as radiation dose, cost effectiveness, and accessibility.[112]

CLINICS CARE POINTS

- Patients at high risk for breast cancer may start mammographic screening earlier than 40 years of age and typically undergo supplemental screening with breast MR imaging
- Patients at intermediate risk for breast cancer may undergo supplemental screening depending on their specific clinical scenario.
- Modalities under consideration for supplemental screening in patients at intermediate risk include DBT, ultrasound examination, CESM, abbreviated or standard diagnostic breast MR imaging, and MBI.
- Dense breasts decrease the sensitivity of mammography for the detection of breast cancer and also increase the risk for developing breast cancer.
- Ultrasound examination detects additional cancers in the setting of increased breast density at a cost of a high-false positive rate.
- Breast MR imaging detects the most breast cancers in all patients, including those with dense breasts, and the recent development of abbreviated examinations may expand the indications for supplemental screening.
- MBI is not recommended for screening at this time given the whole body radiation dose with the intravenous injection of ^{99m}Tc-sestamibi.

DISCLOSURE

L. Wang: No disclosures. R.M. Strigel: Research support, GE Healthcare.

REFERENCES

1. Duffy S, Tabar L, Smith RA. The mammographic screening trials: commentary on the recent work by Olsen and Gotzsche. J Surg Oncol 2002; 81(4):159–62 [discussion: 162–6].

2. Hendrick RE, Baker JA, Helvie MA. Breast cancer deaths averted over 3 decades. Cancer 2019; 125(9):1482–8.

3. Broeders M, Moss S, Nystrom L, et al. The impact of mammographic screening on breast cancer mortality in Europe: a review of observational studies. J Med Screen 2012;19(Suppl 1):14–25.

4. Coldman A, Phillips N, Wilson C, et al. Pan-Canadian study of mammography screening and mortality from breast cancer. J Natl Cancer Inst 2014;106(11).

5. Nickson C, Mason KE, English DR, et al. Mammographic screening and breast cancer mortality: a case-control study and meta-analysis. Cancer Epidemiol Biomarkers Prev 2012;21(9):1479–88.

6. Oeffinger KC, Fontham ET, Etzioni R, et al. Breast cancer screening for women at average risk: 2015 guideline update from the American Cancer Society. JAMA 2015;314(15):1599–614.

7. Tabar L, Yen AM, Wu WY, et al. Insights from the breast cancer screening trials: how screening affects the natural history of breast cancer and implications for evaluating service screening programs. Breast J 2015;21(1):13–20.

8. Rosenberg RD, Hunt WC, Williamson MR, et al. Effects of age, breast density, ethnicity, and estrogen replacement therapy on screening mammographic sensitivity and cancer stage at diagnosis: review of 183,134 screening mammograms in Albuquerque, New Mexico. Radiology 1998;209(2):511–8.

9. Lo G, Scaranelo AM, Aboras H, et al. Evaluation of the utility of screening mammography for high-risk women undergoing screening breast MR imaging. Radiology 2017;285(1):36–43.

10. Narayan AK, Visvanathan K, Harvey SC. Comparative effectiveness of breast MRI and mammography in screening young women with elevated risk of developing breast cancer: a retrospective cohort study. Breast Cancer Res Treat 2016; 158(3):583–9.

11. Passaperuma K, Warner E, Causer PA, et al. Long-term results of screening with magnetic resonance imaging in women with BRCA mutations. Br J Cancer 2012;107(1):24–30.

12. Phi XA, Saadatmand S, De Bock GH, et al. Contribution of mammography to MRI screening in BRCA mutation carriers by BRCA status and age: individual patient data meta-analysis. Br J Cancer 2016; 114(6):631–7.

13. van Zelst JCM, Mus RDM, Woldringh G, et al. Surveillance of women with the BRCA1 or BRCA2 mutation by using biannual automated breast US, MR imaging, and mammography. Radiology 2017; 285(2):376–88.

14. Monticciolo DL, Newell MS, Moy L, et al. Breast cancer screening in women at higher-than-average risk: recommendations from the ACR. J Am Coll Radiol 2018;15:408–15.

15. Elezaby M, Lees B, Maturen KE, et al. BRCA mutation carriers: breast and ovarian cancer screening guidelines and imaging considerations. Radiology 2019;291(3):554–69.

16. Antoniou A, Pharoah PD, Narod S, et al. Average risks of breast and ovarian cancer associated with BRCA1 or BRCA2 mutations detected in case Series unselected for family history: a combined analysis of 22 studies. Am J Hum Genet 2003;72(5):1117–30.

17. Hendrick RE. Radiation doses and risk in breast screening. Journal of Breast Imaging 2020;2(3): 188–200.

18. Genetic/familial high-risk assessment: breast, ovarian, and pancreatic. NCCN Clinical Practice Guidelines in Oncology 2019;Version 1.2020.

19. Saslow D, Boetes C, Burke W, et al. American Cancer Society guidelines for breast screening with MRI as an adjunct to mammography. CA Cancer J Clin 2007;57(2):75–89.

20. Vysotskaia V, Kaseniit KE, Bucheit L, et al. Clinical utility of hereditary cancer panel testing: impact of PALB2, ATM, CHEK2, NBN, BRIP1, RAD51C, and RAD51D results on patient management and adherence to provider recommendations. Cancer 2020;126(3):549–58.

21. Breast Cancer Screening and Diagnosis. NCCN Clinical Practice Guidelines in Oncology. 2019; Version 1.2019.

22. Mulder RL, Kremer LC, Hudson MM, et al. Recommendations for breast cancer surveillance for female survivors of childhood, adolescent, and young adult cancer given chest radiation: a report from the International Late Effects of Childhood Cancer Guideline Harmonization Group. Lancet Oncol 2013;14(13):e621–9.

23. Koo E, Henderson MA, Dwyer M, et al. Management and prevention of breast cancer after radiation to the chest for childhood, adolescent, and young adulthood malignancy. Ann Surg Oncol 2015;22(Suppl 3):S545–51.

24. Mariscotti G, Belli P, Bernardi D, et al. Mammography and MRI for screening women who underwent chest radiation therapy (lymphoma survivors): recommendations for surveillance from the Italian College of Breast Radiologists by SIRM. Radiol Med 2016;121(11):834–7.

25. Lee CH, Dershaw DD, Kopans D, et al. Breast cancer screening with imaging: recommendations from the Society of Breast Imaging and the ACR on the use of mammography, breast MRI, breast ultrasound, and other technologies for the detection of clinically occult breast cancer. J Am Coll Radiol 2010;7(1):18–27.

26. Houssami N, Miglioretti DL. Early detection of breast cancer the second time around:

mammography in women with a personal history of breast cancer. Med J Aust 2011;194(9):439–40.

27. Houssami N, Abraham LA, Miglioretti DL, et al. Accuracy and outcomes of screening mammography in women with a personal history of early-stage breast cancer. JAMA 2011;305(8): 790–9.

28. Arpino G, Laucirica R, Elledge RM. Premalignant and in situ breast disease: biology and clinical implications. Ann Intern Med 2005;143(6):446–57.

29. Dupont WD, Page DL. Risk factors for breast cancer in women with proliferative breast disease. N Engl J Med 1985;312(3):146–51.

30. D'Orsi CJ, Sickles E, Mendelson EB, et al. ACR BI-RADS atlas, breast imaging reporting and data system. Reston (VA): American College of Radiology; 2013.

31. Tice JA, Kerlikowske K. Supplemental breast cancer screening: a density conundrum. J Gen Intern Med 2017;32(6):593–4.

32. Boyd NF, Byng JW, Jong RA, et al. Quantitative classification of mammographic densities and breast cancer risk: results from the Canadian National Breast Screening Study. J Natl Cancer Inst 1995;87(9):670–5.

33. Boyd NF, Guo H, Martin LJ, et al. Mammographic density and the risk and detection of breast cancer. N Engl J Med 2007;356(3):227–36.

34. Boyd NF, Martin LJ, Sun L, et al. Body size, mammographic density, and breast cancer risk. Cancer Epidemiol biomarkers Prev 2006;15(11): 2086–92.

35. Byrne C, Schairer C, Wolfe J, et al. Mammographic features and breast cancer risk: effects with time, age, and menopause status. J Natl Cancer Inst 1995;87(21):1622–9.

36. Ursin G, Ma H, Wu AH, et al. Mammographic density and breast cancer in three ethnic groups. Cancer Epidemiol biomarkers Prev 2003;12(4):332–8.

37. Vacek PM, Geller BM. A prospective study of breast cancer risk using routine mammographic breast density measurements. Cancer Epidemiol biomarkers Prev 2004;13(5):715–22.

38. Sickles EA. The use of breast imaging to screen women at high risk for cancer. Radiol Clin North Am 2010;48(5):859–78.

39. Boyd NF, Martin LJ, Bronskill M, et al. Breast tissue composition and susceptibility to breast cancer. J Natl Cancer Inst 2010;102(16):1224–37.

40. McCormack VA, dos Santos Silva I. Breast density and parenchymal patterns as markers of breast cancer risk: a meta-analysis. Cancer Epidemiol biomarkers Prev 2006;15(6):1159–69.

41. Destounis SV, Santacroce A, Arieno A. Update on breast density, risk estimation, and supplemental screening. AJR Am J Roentgenol 2020;214(2): 296–305.

42. Rafferty EA, Durand MA, Conant EF, et al. Breast cancer screening using tomosynthesis and digital mammography in dense and nondense breasts. JAMA 2016;315(16):1784–6.

43. Vedantham S, Karellas A, Vijayaraghavan GR, et al. Digital breast tomosynthesis: state of the art. Radiology 2015;277(3):663–84.

44. Sujlana PS, Mahesh M, Vedantham S, et al. Digital breast tomosynthesis: image acquisition principles and artifacts. Clin Imaging 2019;55:188–95.

45. Ciatto S, Houssami N, Bernardi D, et al. Integration of 3D digital mammography with tomosynthesis for population breast-cancer screening (STORM): a prospective comparison study. Lancet Oncol 2013;14(7):583–9.

46. Skaane P, Bandos AI, Gullien R, et al. Comparison of digital mammography alone and digital mammography plus tomosynthesis in a population-based screening program. Radiology 2013;267(1):47–56.

47. Friedewald SM, Rafferty EA, Rose SL, et al. Breast cancer screening using tomosynthesis in combination with digital mammography. JAMA 2014; 311(24):2499–507.

48. Haas BM, Kalra V, Geisel J, et al. Comparison of tomosynthesis plus digital mammography and digital mammography alone for breast cancer screening. Radiology 2013;269(3):694–700.

49. Sia J, Moodie K, Bressel M, et al. A prospective study comparing digital breast tomosynthesis with digital mammography in surveillance after breast cancer treatment. Eur J Cancer 2016;61: 122–7.

50. Maxwell AJ, Michell M, Lim YY, et al. A randomised trial of screening with digital breast tomosynthesis plus conventional digital 2D mammography versus 2D mammography alone in younger higher risk women. Eur J Radiol 2017;94:133–9.

51. Pisano ED. Is Tomosynthesis the Future of Breast Cancer Screening? Radiology 2018;287(1):47–8.

52. Houssami N, Turner RM. Rapid review: estimates of incremental breast cancer detection from tomosynthesis (3D-mammography) screening in women with dense breasts. Breast 2016;30:141–5.

53. Tice JAO, Ollendorf DA, Lee JM, et al. The comparative clinical effectiveness and value of supplemental screening tests following negative mammography in women with dense breast tissue. The New England Comparative Effectiveness Public Advisory Council Public Meeting Proceeding. Institute for Clinical and Economic Review. Boston, MA, December 13, 2013.

54. Melnikow J, Fenton JJ, Whitlock EP, et al. Supplemental screening for breast cancer in women with dense breasts: a systematic review for the U.S. Preventive Services Task Force. Ann Intern Med 2016;164(4):268–78.

55. Tagliafico AS, Calabrese M, Mariscotti G, et al. Adjunct screening with tomosynthesis or ultrasound in women with mammography-negative dense breasts: interim report of a prospective comparative trial. J Clin Oncol 2016;34(16): 1882–8.

56. Tagliafico AS, Mariscotti G, Valdora F, et al. A prospective comparative trial of adjunct screening with tomosynthesis or ultrasound in women with mammography-negative dense breasts (ASTOUND-2). Eur J Cancer 2018;104: 39–46.

57. Expert Panel on Breast Imaging, Mainiero MB, Moy L, Baron P, et al. ACR appropriateness criteria((r)) breast cancer screening. J Am Coll Radiol 2017;14(11S):S383–90.

58. Covington MF, Pizzitola VJ, Lorans R, et al. The future of contrast-enhanced mammography. AJR Am J Roentgenol 2018;210(2):292–300.

59. Tagliafico AS, Bignotti B, Rossi F, et al. Diagnostic performance of contrast-enhanced spectral mammography: systematic review and meta-analysis. Breast 2016;28:13–9.

60. Mori M, Akashi-Tanaka S, Suzuki S, et al. Diagnostic accuracy of contrast-enhanced spectral mammography in comparison to conventional full-field digital mammography in a population of women with dense breasts. Breast Cancer 2017; 24(1):104–10.

61. Jochelson MS, Pinker K, Dershaw DD, et al. Comparison of screening CEDM and MRI for women at increased risk for breast cancer: a pilot study. Eur J Radiol 2017;97:37–43.

62. Sorin V, Yagil Y, Yosepovich A, et al. Contrast-enhanced spectral mammography in women with intermediate breast cancer risk and dense breasts. AJR Am J Roentgenol 2018;211(5):W267–74.

63. Sung JS, Lebron L, Keating D, et al. Performance of dual-energy contrast-enhanced digital mammography for screening women at increased risk of breast cancer. Radiology 2019;293(1):81–8.

64. Vourtsis A, Berg WA. Breast density implications and supplemental screening. Eur Radiol 2019; 29(4):1762–77.

65. Ohuchi N, Suzuki A, Sobue T, et al. Sensitivity and specificity of mammography and adjunctive ultrasonography to screen for breast cancer in the Japan Strategic Anti-cancer Randomized Trial (J-START): a randomised controlled trial. Lancet 2016;387(10016):341–8.

66. Kim SY, Han BK, Kim EK, et al. Breast Cancer Detected at Screening US: survival rates and clinical-pathologic and imaging factors associated with recurrence. Radiology 2017;284(2): 354–64.

67. Kuhl C, Weigel S, Schrading S, et al. Prospective multicenter cohort study to refine management

recommendations for women at elevated familial risk of breast cancer: the EVA trial. J Clin Oncol 2010;28(9):1450–7.

68. Kuhl CK, Schrading S, Leutner CC, et al. Mammography, breast ultrasound, and magnetic resonance imaging for surveillance of women at high familial risk for breast cancer. J Clin Oncol 2005;23(33): 8469–76.

69. Sardanelli F, Podo F, Santoro F, et al. Multicenter surveillance of women at high genetic breast cancer risk using mammography, ultrasonography, and contrast-enhanced magnetic resonance imaging (the High Breast Cancer Risk Italian 1 Study): final results. Invest Radiol 2011;46(2): 94–105.

70. Berg WA, Blume JD, Cormack JB, et al. Combined screening with ultrasound and mammography vs mammography alone in women at elevated risk of breast cancer. JAMA 2008;299(18):2151–63.

71. Berg WA, Zhang Z, Lehrer D, et al. Detection of breast cancer with addition of annual screening ultrasound or a single screening MRI to mammography in women with elevated breast cancer risk. JAMA 2012;307(13):1394–404.

72. Hooley RJ, Greenberg KL, Stackhouse RM, et al. Screening US in patients with mammographically dense breasts: initial experience with Connecticut Public Act 09-41. Radiology 2012;265(1):59–69.

73. Weigert J, Steenbergen S. The Connecticut experiment: the role of ultrasound in the screening of women with dense breasts. Breast J 2012;18(6): 517–22.

74. Dibble EH, Singer TM, Jimoh N, et al. Dense breast ultrasound screening after digital mammography versus after digital breast tomosynthesis. AJR Am J Roentgenol 2019;213(6):1397–402.

75. Berg WA, Blume JD, Cormack JB, et al. Operator dependence of physician-performed whole-breast US: lesion detection and characterization. Radiology 2006;241(2):355–65.

76. Rebolj M, Assi V, Brentnall A, et al. Addition of ultrasound to mammography in the case of dense breast tissue: systematic review and meta-analysis. Br J Cancer 2018;118(12):1559–70.

77. Crystal P, Strano SD, Shcharynski S, et al. Using sonography to screen women with mammographically dense breasts. AJR Am J Roentgenol 2003; 181(1):177–82.

78. Kaplan SS. Clinical utility of bilateral whole-breast US in the evaluation of women with dense breast tissue. Radiology 2001;221(3):641–9.

79. Kelly KM, Dean J, Comulada WS, et al. Breast cancer detection using automated whole breast ultrasound and mammography in radiographically dense breasts. Eur Radiol 2010;20(3):734–42.

80. Brem RF, Tabar L, Duffy SW, et al. Assessing improvement in detection of breast cancer with three-dimensional automated breast US in women with dense breast tissue: the SomoInsight Study. Radiology 2015;274(3):663–73.

81. Wilczek B, Wilczek HE, Rasouliyan L, et al. Adding 3D automated breast ultrasound to mammography screening in women with heterogeneously and extremely dense breasts: report from a hospital-based, high-volume, single-center breast cancer screening program. Eur J Radiol 2016;85(9): 1554–63.

82. Sprague BL, Stout NK, Schechter C, et al. Benefits, harms, and cost-effectiveness of supplemental ultrasonography screening for women with dense breasts. Ann Intern Med 2015;162(3): 157–66.

83. Mann RM, Cho N, Moy L. Breast MRI: state of the art. Radiology 2019;292(3):520–36.

84. Kriege M, Brekelmans CT, Boetes C, et al. Efficacy of MRI and mammography for breast-cancer screening in women with a familial or genetic predisposition. N Engl J Med 2004;351(5):427–37.

85. Leach MO, Boggis CR, Dixon AK, et al. Screening with magnetic resonance imaging and mammography of a UK population at high familial risk of breast cancer: a prospective multicentre cohort study (MARIBS). Lancet 2005; 365(9473):1769–78.

86. Rijnsburger AJ, Obdeijn IM, Kaas R, et al. BRCA1-associated breast cancers present differently from BRCA2-associated and familial cases: long-term follow-up of the Dutch MRISC Screening Study. J Clin Oncol 2010;28(36):5265–73.

87. Freitas V, Scaranelo A, Menezes R, et al. Added cancer yield of breast magnetic resonance imaging screening in women with a prior history of chest radiation therapy. Cancer 2013;119(3):495–503.

88. Ng AK, Garber JE, Diller LR, et al. Prospective study of the efficacy of breast magnetic resonance imaging and mammographic screening in survivors of Hodgkin lymphoma. J Clin Oncol 2013; 31(18):2282–8.

89. Sung JS, Lee CH, Morris EA, et al. Screening breast MR imaging in women with a history of chest irradiation. Radiology 2011;259(1):65–71.

90. Tieu MT, Cigsar C, Ahmed S, et al. Breast cancer detection among young survivors of pediatric Hodgkin lymphoma with screening magnetic resonance imaging. Cancer 2014;120(16):2507–13.

91. Brennan S, Liberman L, Dershaw DD, et al. Breast MRI screening of women with a personal history of breast cancer. AJR Am J Roentgenol 2010;195(2): 510–6.

92. Giess CS, Poole PS, Chikarmane SA, et al. Screening Breast MRI in patients previously treated for breast cancer: diagnostic yield for cancer and abnormal interpretation rate. Acad Radiol 2015; 22(11):1331–7.

93. Gweon HM, Cho N, Han W, et al. Breast MR imaging screening in women with a history of breast conservation therapy. Radiology 2014;272(2): 366–73.

94. Lehman CD, Lee JM, DeMartini WB, et al. Screening MRI in women with a personal history of breast cancer. J Natl Cancer Inst 2016;108(3): djv349.

95. Schacht DV, Yamaguchi K, Lai J, et al. Importance of a personal history of breast cancer as a risk factor for the development of subsequent breast cancer: results from screening breast MRI. AJR Am J Roentgenol 2014;202(2):289–92.

96. Strigel RM, Rollenhagen J, Burnside ES, et al. Screening breast MRI outcomes in routine clinical practice: comparison to BI-RADS benchmarks. Acad Radiol 2017;24(4):411–7.

97. Weinstock C, Campassi C, Goloubeva O, et al. Breast magnetic resonance imaging (MRI) surveillance in breast cancer survivors. Springerplus 2015;4:459.

98. Wernli KJ, Ichikawa L, Kerlikowske K, et al. Surveillance breast MRI and mammography: comparison in women with a personal history of breast cancer. Radiology 2019;292(2):311–8.

99. Friedlander LC, Roth SO, Gavenonis SC. Results of MR imaging screening for breast cancer in high-risk patients with lobular carcinoma in situ. Radiology 2011;261(2):421–7.

100. Sung JS, Malak SF, Bajaj P, et al. Screening breast MR imaging in women with a history of lobular carcinoma in situ. Radiology 2011;261(2):414–20.

101. Bakker MF, de Lange SV, Pijnappel RM, et al. Supplemental MRI screening for women with extremely dense breast tissue. N Engl J Med 2019;381(22): 2091–102.

102. Comstock CE, Gatsonis C, Newstead GM, et al. Comparison of Abbreviated Breast MRI vs digital breast tomosynthesis for breast cancer detection among women with dense breasts undergoing screening. JAMA 2020;323(8):746–56.

103. Hruska CB. Molecular breast imaging for screening in dense breasts: state of the art and future directions. AJR Am J Roentgenol 2017;208(2):275–83.

104. Sun Y, Wei W, Yang HW, et al. Clinical usefulness of breast-specific gamma imaging as an adjunct modality to mammography for diagnosis of breast cancer: a systemic review and meta-analysis. Eur J Nucl Med Mol Imaging 2013;40(3):450–63.

105. Rhodes DJ, Hruska CB, Conners AL, et al. Journal club: molecular breast imaging at reduced radiation dose for supplemental screening in mammographically dense breasts. AJR Am J Roentgenol 2015;204(2):241–51.

106. Rhodes DJ, Hruska CB, Phillips SW, et al. Dedicated dual-head gamma imaging for breast cancer screening in women with mammographically dense breasts. Radiology 2011;258(1):106–18.

107. Brem RF, Ruda RC, Yang JL, et al. Breast-specific gamma-imaging for the detection of mammographically occult breast cancer in women at increased risk. J Nucl Med 2016;57(5):678–84.

108. Huppe AI, Mehta AK, Brem RF. Molecular breast imaging: a comprehensive review. Semin Ultrasound CT MR 2018;39(1):60–9.

109. Tao AT, Hruska CB, Conners AL, et al. Dose reduction in molecular breast imaging with a new image-processing algorithm. AJR Am J Roentgenol 2020; 214(1):185–93.

110. Breast Cancer. NCCN Clinical Practice Guidelines in Oncology. 2020;Version 3.2020.

111. Committee opinion no. 625: management of women with dense breasts diagnosed by mammography. Obstet Gynecol 2015;125(3): 750–1.

112. Fowler AM. Molecular imaging approaches for supplemental screening in women at increased breast cancer risk. J Nucl Med 2016;57(5):661–2.

113. Genetic/Familial High-Risk Assessment: Colorectal. NCCN Clinical Practice Guidelines in Oncology. 2019;Version 3.2019.

114. ACR manual on contrast media. Available at: https://www.acr.org/-/media/ACR/Files/Clinical-Resources/Contrast_Media.pdf. Accessed May 13, 2020.

Magnetic Resonance Imaging in Screening of Breast Cancer

Yiming Gao, MD[a],*, Beatriu Reig, MD, MPH[a], Laura Heacock, MS, MD[a], Debbie L. Bennett, MD[b], Samantha L. Heller, PhD, MD[a], Linda Moy, MD[a,c,d]

KEYWORDS

- Magnetic resonance imaging • Breast cancer screening • Abbreviated MR imaging
- High-risk screening • Supplemental screening

KEY POINTS

- Magnetic resonance (MR) imaging has a modality-based advantage compared to mammography and sonography in early detection of invasive breast cancer, which is being leveraged to optimize screening outcomes.
- Supplemental screening with MR imaging has been found to be of value in high-risk women as well as in certain subgroups of higher-than-average-risk women, but careful cost-benefit considerations are needed.
- Overall adherence to MR imaging among currently eligible women is poor even as screening indications of MR imaging continue to evolve.

INTRODUCTION

Magnetic resonance (MR) imaging is an advanced modality currently reserved for supplemental breast cancer screening in high-risk individuals, with excellent sensitivity and specificity reported in recent literature.[1-5] Although MR imaging–specific impact on breast cancer mortality is difficult to assess, supplemental screening with MR imaging has been associated with detection of earlier-stage disease and improved 10-year survival.[6,7] Although mammography is the standard of care for population-wide screening known to decrease mortality, questions of overdiagnosis and overtreatment persist.[8] With increasingly sophisticated understanding of breast cancer heterogeneity and outcomes based on cancer subtypes, there is growing impetus to parse out modality-based cancer yield both in number and

in the type of cancers detected. The advantage of contrast-enhanced MR imaging as a functional imaging modality optimized to capture biologically more aggressive tumors that may be mammographically occult is the basis of a growing interest in expanding the role of MR imaging in breast cancer screening. Furthermore, there is growing evidence that MR imaging also outperforms mammography and sonography in moderate-risk women in cancer yield, prompting more recent broadening of MR imaging screening indications in certain guidelines.[9] However, patient access to MR imaging remains limited, and the cost and time currently associated with the examination can be prohibitive. Efforts to improve feasibility of wider implementation have focused on streamlining examination acquisition and interpretation while preserving diagnostic accuracy. This article therefore (1) provides an evidence-based overview

This work has not received grant funding.
[a] Department of Radiology, NYU School of Medicine, 160 East 34th Street, New York, NY 10016, USA;
[b] Department of Radiology, Washington University School of Medicine, 510 S. Kingshighway, Box 8131, St Louis, MO 63110, USA; [c] Department of Radiology, NYU Center for Biomedical Imaging, 660 First Avenue, New York, NY 10016, USA; [d] Department of Radiology, NYU Center for Advanced Imaging Innovation and Research, 660 First Avenue, New York, NY 10016, USA
* Corresponding author. 160 East 34th Street, New York, NY 10016.
E-mail address: yiming.gao@nyulangone.org

Radiol Clin N Am 59 (2021) 85–98
https://doi.org/10.1016/j.rcl.2020.09.004

of current MR imaging screening indications, (2) considers the rationale for expanding its use in the population, and (3) discusses challenges and potential solutions in improving its cost-effectiveness with abbreviated approaches, notably via abbreviated and ultrafast MR imaging protocols.

CURRENT MAGNETIC RESONANCE IMAGING SCREENING INDICATIONS
High-Risk Screening

Women with an estimated lifetime risk (LTR) of greater than or equal to 20% to 25% for developing breast cancer are defined as high risk as per the American Cancer Society (ACS) guidelines.[10] A woman's LTR is usually estimated based on family history and risk modeling algorithms. There is well-established evidence supporting MR imaging screening in this group,[11–13] for whom annual supplemental MR imaging in addition to mammography is currently the standard of care in breast cancer screening.

Hereditary and Familial Risks

Although there are variations in what constitutes high risk across multidisciplinary guidelines, BRCA germline mutation carriers and untested first-degree relatives are universally acknowledged as harboring risks an order of magnitude greater than that of the general population, and are thought to benefit the most from MR imaging screening[9,10,14–20](see Table 2). Pooled data have shown that the average risk of developing breast cancer by age 70 years is 65% for BRCA1 mutation carriers and 45% for BRCA2 mutation carriers.[21] Compared with women without mutations, BRCA1 and BRCA2 carriers have, on average, respectively 30-fold and 10-fold to 16-fold higher LTR of breast cancer.[21] In women with BRCA mutations who undergo screening, mammography has low sensitivity because of high breast density and more rapidly growing tumors in younger women.[6] Prospective trials have shown that annual supplemental MR imaging in conjunction with mammography typically doubles the sensitivity of mammography alone and generally achieves sensitivities greater than 90%.[3,4,11,13,22,23] Further ultrasonography or clinical breast examination are not additive[24](Table 1). False-positive rates are increased with addition of screening MR imaging to annual mammography, but these false-positives tend to decrease in successive incident rounds of screening. In a multicentered prospective trial from the Netherlands, the sensitivity advantage of MR imaging versus mammography was greatest at prevalent round (93% vs 20%; P = .003) but

maintained in subsequent rounds (77% vs 29%; P = .02); and the false-positive rate of MR imaging decreased in subsequent rounds (from 14% to 8%).[25] MR imaging–detected cancers also have a favorable stage distribution in BRCA mutation carriers, primarily composed of sub–1-cm invasive cancers and in situ cancers at incident rounds of screening with low rates of node positivity (12%–26%), associated with improved 10-year survival.[24] Importantly, timing the frequency of screening has been a challenge in this population. Particularly in BRCA1 carriers less than 50 years of age, who are known to have the highest rate of interval cancers because of a high prevalence of rapidly growing tumors, annual imaging may not be adequate.[26–28] The main strategy has been to shorten the screening interval to every 6 months using various examination combinations, such as staggering mammography and MR imaging, or using biannual MR imaging with annual mammography, or by supplementing annual mammography/MR imaging with biannual ultrasonography.[23,29] MR imaging screening is generally deemed cost-effective for BRCA carriers assuming perfect attendance, particular for BRCA1 carriers, and adherence to the examination is high among carriers confirmed by genetic testing (80%–90%).[30,31]

Annual breast MR imaging is also recommended in less common mutations associated with high risk of breast cancer, such as TP53 (Li-Fraumeni syndrome; 95% by age 90 years) and PTEN (Bannayan-Riley-Ruvalcaba syndrome, Cowden syndrome; 85% by age 80 years), and is increasingly considered in additional mutations associated with moderate to high risk of breast cancer, including CDH1, STK11, PALB2, CHEK2, ATM, BARD1, and NF1, with individual decisions often guided by family history because of a further increased risk.[32–36] However, most women with a family history of breast cancer do not have an identified genetic mutation, and 15% of all breast cancers occur in this group.[37,38] Family history in these women therefore serves as the primary basis for calculating LTR via modeling algorithms, and is a direct indication for supplemental MR imaging screening if calculated risk exceeds 20%.[10] In this group, MR imaging has been found to increase detection of early-stage cancer compared with mammography (14 per 1000 vs 5 per 1000 cancers; P<.0003).[12] Notably, in contrast with BRCA carriers, women at high risk without BRCA mutations have been found to have significantly lower adherence to supplemental screening MR imaging.[39,40] There is also evidence that, although supplemental MR imaging is underused in high-risk women, many who undergo breast MR

Table 1
Comparison of diagnostic performance using magnetic resonance imaging versus mammography or sonography in multimodality breast cancer screening among high-risk women based on outcomes of prospective studies

Reference	Patients (n)	Rounds (n)[a]	Inclusion	Sensitivity			Specificity			PPV3			Interval CA (n)
				MR Imaging (%)	MG (%)	US (%)	MR Imaging (%)	MG (%)	US (%)	MR Imaging (%)	MG (%)	US (%)	
2020[11]	8782	20,053	BRCA+/Fam	91	41	NA	87	92	NA	20	26	NA	12
2019[12],[b]	674	2812	Fam	98	87	NA	84	91	NA	27	28	NA	1
2017[13]	296	1170	BRCA+/Fam	68	37	32	95	98	95	25	34	10	3
2015[22]	559	1506	BRCA+/Fam	90	38	38	89	97	97	20	28	27	1
2014[23]	221	1855	BRCA+	100	27	77	56	82	84	NA	NA	NA	1
2012[26]	612	612	Mixed/Dense	88	52	45	76	91	90	23	38	12	9
2011[3]	501	1592	BRCA+/Fam	91	50	52	97	99	98	56	71	62	3
2010[4]	687	1679	BRCA+/Fam	93	33	37	98	99	98	48	39	36	0

All studies included are prospective in design.

Abbreviations: BRCA+, BRCA1 or BRCA2 mutation carriers; Interval CA, interval cancers after all-modality screening; Fam, familial risk for breast cancer as defined by a calculated lifetime risk of breast cancer greater than or equal to 20%; NA, not available; PPV3, positive predictive value indicating the rate of positive biopsies among biopsied lesions.

[a] Number of rounds of screening indicates rounds that specifically include MR imaging.

[b] Randomized controlled study comparing MR imaging versus mammography.

imaging may not be appropriately high risk.[41,42] For example, for those with family history who undergo multigene panel testing in recent years, unclassified genetic variations of uncertain significance (VUS) are increasingly encountered. Although work is being done to better classify these genetic variants to provide clinically actionable information, detection of any unknown variant (including BRCA1/2 VUS) is currently not an indication for intensified breast cancer screening.[43]

Prior Chest Radiation

Women with prior childhood chest radiation are another group at high risk for developing breast cancer later in life, for whom annual screening MR imaging is consistently recommended (**Table 2**). By age 50 years of age, 1 in 3 women with prior chest radiation (risk greatest if subjected to ≥20 Gy) are diagnosed with breast cancer, a risk on par with that of BRCA1 mutation carriers.[44,45] Multiple studies have shown increased sensitivity of both mammography and MR imaging in this group (94%–100%), with supplemental MR imaging yielding additional cancers.[46–48] Therefore, annual screening mammography and breast MR imaging are recommended, starting at age 25 years or 8 years following chest radiation, whichever occurs last.[10] However, breast cancer screening adherence among childhood cancer survivors is poor. Notably, mammography screening adherence in women who have received chest radiation is lower than among their average-risk peers in the general population. Nearly half of survivors younger than 40 years of age have never obtained a mammogram, and only 52% of women aged 40 to 50 years undergo regular mammography screening.[49–51] Adherence for MR imaging screening is markedly worse, and efforts to improve adherence have had marginal effects. In a recent randomized controlled study, although educational interventions increased the rate of uptake of mammography screening (from 18% to 33%), MR imaging uptake was not significantly changed (from 13% to 16%), and overall screening adherence in this population remains poor. Primary barriers identified by women survivors to completing screening included lack of physician recommendation, deferred action by survivor, absence of symptoms, and cost, which is a concern specific to MR imaging.[51]

EVOLVING MAGNETIC RESONANCE IMAGING SCREENING INDICATIONS
Moderate-Risk Screening

Despite a lack of consensus among different guidelines, there is increasing evidence supporting expanding the indications of MR imaging screening to include women at intermediate risk for breast cancer, as defined by an estimated LTR of 15% to 20% as per the ACS.[10] In particular, several subgroups of women with higher-than-average risk for breast cancer are considered, including those with a personal history of breast cancer, dense breast tissue, or a history of atypical epithelial hyperplasia (atypical ductal hyperplasia [ADH], atypical lobular hyperplasia [ALH], and lobular carcinoma in situ [LCIS]). Although the 2007 ACS guidelines reported insufficient evidence to recommend for or against MR imaging screening in these groups, the more recent 2018 American College of Radiology (ACR) and 2020 National Comprehensive Cancer Network (NCCN) guidelines suggest considering MR imaging in some or all of these women, particularly in conjunction with other overlapping risk factors that may increase LTR to greater than 20% (see **Table 2**).

Breast Cancer Survivors

Women with a personal history of breast cancer are at considerable risk of developing a second breast cancer, with cumulative risks estimated at 5.4% in 5 years and 19.3% in 10 years following initial diagnosis.[52,53] In women diagnosed with breast cancer before age 50 years, the LTR for a second breast cancer is greater than 20%.[54] Additional independent predictors of increased risk for a second breast cancer within 5 years also include aggressive tumor biology in the first cancer, treatment without radiation, and heterogeneously dense breasts on mammography.[52] Therefore, the ACR Appropriateness Criteria currently recommend annual screening MR imaging in conjunction with mammography for women with breast cancer diagnosed before age 50 years, and for women with breast cancer history and dense breasts.[9] Mammographic sensitivity is limited in the treated breast because of postsurgical parenchymal distortion, scarring, and fat necrosis. Although there are currently no prospective data, a growing body of retrospective studies have consistently shown superior sensitivities using MR imaging compared with mammography in women with a personal history of breast cancer (80%–100% vs 0%–53%),[55,56] and supplemental MR imaging in this group has been shown to perform as well as, if not better than, in those with genetic and familial predispositions[57] (**Fig. 1**). The 2018 ACR recommendations aim to optimize early detection of second breast cancers and improve survival but have not been universally adopted across multidisciplinary guidelines, pending data on mortality benefits, which are currently unknown (see **Table 2**).

Table 2
Multidisciplinary recommendations for annual supplemental magnetic resonance imaging screening in higher-than-average-risk women

Organization	BRCA Carriers/First-Degree Relatives[a]	Family History	Prior Radiation	Personal History	Dense Tissue	History of Atypia[b]
ACS 2007	BRCA1/2/select mutations	If LTR ≥20%	Age 10–30 y	NR	NR	NR
ACR 2018	BRCA1/2/select mutations	If LTR ≥20%	Age<30 y	If early diagnosis (before age 50)	If personal history (prior breast cancer)	If other risk factors
ASBrS 2019	BRCA1/2/select mutations	If strong family history	Age 10–30 y	If early diagnosis (before age 50 y)	If personal history (prior breast cancer)	NR
NCCN 2020	BRCA1/2/select mutations	If family history suggests hereditary pattern despite absence of mutation (eg, early diagnosis before age 30 y)	Age<30 y	NR	NR	If LTR ≥20%
EUSOBI 2015	BRCA1/2/select mutations	Selective	Age<30 y	NR	NR	NR
ECIBS 2020[c]	NS	NR	NS	NS	NR	NR
ACOG 2017	BRCA1/2/select mutations	If LTR ≥20%	Age 10–30 y	If other risks	NR	NR

Abbreviations: ACR, American College of Radiology; ASBrS, American Society of Breast Surgeons; ECIBS, European Commission Initiative on Breast Cancer; EUSOBI, European Society of Breast Imaging; NCCN, National Comprehensive Cancer Network; NR, screening not recommended or insufficient evidence to recommend for or against; NS, not specified.
[a] MR imaging is consistently recommended for *BRCA* mutation carriers and untested first-degree relatives, but more variably recommended or considered for other mutations.
[b] Atypia refers to atypical epithelial hyperplasia, including atypical lobular hyperplasia, lobular carcinoma in situ, and atypical ductal hyperplasia.
[c] The ECIBS guidelines primarily address average-risk women that attend organized screening programs in Europe but also include select higher-than-average-risk groups such as those with family history or high breast tissue density.

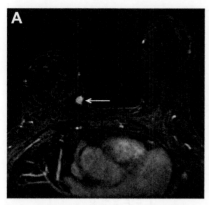 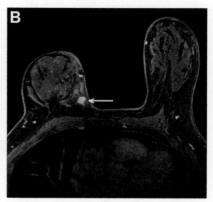 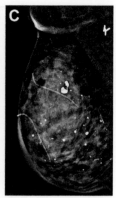

Fig. 1. A 73-year-old woman with dense breast tissue and a prior history of right breast cancer treated with lumpectomy and radiotherapy 6 years prior, found to have a small recurrent invasive ductal carcinoma in the medial posterior right breast on MR imaging, as shown here on axial T1W postcontrast subtraction (*A*) and nonsubtraction (*B*) images (*arrows*). This mass was mammographically occult on the same-day surveillance mammogram (*C*).

Extremely Dense Tissue

Women with extremely dense breast tissue not only have poor sensitivity on mammography (on the order of 61%–65%)[58,59] but also have inherently increased risk for breast cancer (approximately double the average risk)[60] (**Fig. 2**). Clinical presentation of interval cancers following a negative mammogram is 18 times more likely in women with extremely dense breasts than in women with fatty breasts, a statistic that underscores the importance of supplemental imaging in this group.[61] Although digital breast tomosynthesis (DBT) has improved both sensitivity and specificity of cancer detection, it has had minimal benefit in the extremely dense subgroup.[62,63] Breast MR imaging has the highest sensitivity for cancer detection and is not limited by breast density.[64] However, ultrasonography is currently more commonly used in supplemental screening because of wider availability and lower cost of implementation, although its cost-effectiveness has been questioned given the small additional cancer yield.[65] In comparison, MR imaging significantly outperforms ultrasonography in incremental cancer yield (3–4 per 1000 vs 15 per 1000) and has a lower false-positive rate compared with ultrasonography,[66] suggesting MR imaging may be the better supplemental screening method for women with dense breasts. Since 2019, a federal law has been introduced in the United States that mandates the US Food and Drug Administration to develop standardized breast density notification language, which is the first step in paving the way for a more standardized supplemental imaging regimen in dense women.[67]

The Dutch DENSE trial is the first and largest randomized controlled trial to date, evaluating women with extremely dense breast tissue on mammography (as per quantitative volumetric assessment), who are randomized to undergo mammography screening with or without

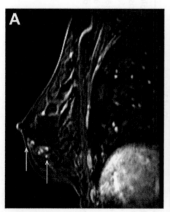 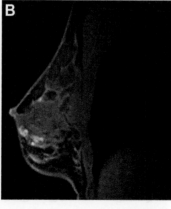

Fig. 2. A 31-year-old woman with *BRCA1* mutation and extremely dense breast tissue with segmental distribution of clumped non–mass enhancement identified on MR imaging screening without mammographic correlate, as shown on sagittal postcontrast T1W subtraction image (*A*) (*arrows*), with subsequent biopsy yielding intermediate-grade to high-grade ductal carcinoma in situ. This finding was mammographically occult and the disease blends in with dense fibroglandular tissue, as shown on the corresponding sagittal postcontrast T1W image (*B*).

supplemental MR imaging (n = 40,373) (age, 50–75 years). The prevalent round screening results with 2-year follow-up showed that supplemental MR imaging screening not only yielded an additional 16.5 per 1000 cancers but was also associated with a 50% reduction in interval cancer rate, suggesting a potential mortality benefit.[68] The ECOG-ACRIN 1141 trial, early results were similarly positive. In this prospective study comparing performance of DBT versus abbreviated MR imaging (ABMR) among women with dense breasts (heterogeneously and extremely dense) (n = 1444; age, 40–75 years), ABMR detected significantly more invasive cancers than DBT (11.8 per 1000 vs 4.8 per 1000), with no interval cancers observed during follow-up.[69] Results for incident rounds of screening are currently pending for both studies, which will help further inform how MR imaging may best be used in women with dense breast tissue.

Atypical Epithelial Hyperplasia

Atypical epithelial hyperplasia refers to a spectrum of proliferative epithelial lesions that are nonobligate precursors to malignancy and are also biological indicators for future increased risk for developing breast cancer. Women with atypical epithelial hyperplasia such as ADH, ALH, and LCIS have a 3 to 10 times higher relative risk for breast cancer than the general population.[70,71] Although these women are currently classified in the intermediate-risk category as per the 2007 ACS guidelines (stated as associated with 15%–20% LTR), more recent data with long-term follow-up indicate this population has an LTR greater than 20%, more consistent with high-risk classification, for which annual MR imaging would be recommended. In longitudinal studies including nearly 1000 women from the Mayo Benign Breast Disease Cohort and the Nashville Breast Cohort, 20% to 30% developed breast cancer on average 12 to 25 years following initial detection of atypical epithelial hyperplasia.[72,73] Women with ADH, ALH, and LCIS are prone to developing higher-grade invasive tumors, and those who undergo mammography screening have a significantly higher interval cancer rate compared with the general population (2.6 per 1000 vs 0.9 per 1000; $P = .002$).[73,74] For these reasons, adjunct screening with MR imaging may add value in this population, given its potential to decrease interval cancers as well as to increase detection of more aggressive disease based on more robust data in other populations. The ACR and NCCN currently both recommend consideration of supplemental MR imaging in women with a history of atypical epithelial hyperplasia, particularly if other risk factors such as family history coexist and if cumulative LTR exceeds 20% (see Table 2). However, current evidence for supplemental MR imaging screening in this population is limited and more data are needed.

Average-Risk Screening

Breast MR imaging screening is currently not recommended in average-risk women (LTR<15% as per the ACS). Although mammography screening has been highly effective in early cancer detection in average-risk women more than 40 years of age, interval cancers persist at a rate of 13% to 38%.[75,76] In contrast, more recent controversies regarding mammography have centered on detection of low-grade disease, which may contribute to overdiagnosis. Functional advantage of MR imaging in preferentially detecting the more aggressive spectrum of disease may be a potential answer to overcoming the shortcomings of mammography. Therefore, MR imaging screening is now beginning to be considered in the average-risk population.

A prospective study of supplemental MR imaging in average-risk women with negative mammography and ultrasonography examinations (n = 2120) found an overall incremental cancer detection rate (CDR) of 15.5 per 1000, which is highly comparable with incremental cancer yield by MR imaging in high-risk women (CDR of 10–20 per 1000).[2,77,78] Importantly, MR imaging–detected cancers in the study were small (median, 8 mm), frequently high grade (46%), and largely node negative (93.4%), with no interval cancers observed.[2] This increased sensitivity for smaller node-negative invasive cancers at MR imaging compared with mammography (average size at detection, 8 mm vs 1–2 cm) and the decreased interval cancer rate suggest a potential to downstage disease and further improve breast cancer–specific survival.[4,77,79] In the study by Kuhl and colleagues,[2] the zero interval cancer rate in the context of a substantial decrease in incremental CDR from prevalent round to incident round screening (22.6 per 1000 to 6.9 per 1000) supports a likely stage shift in cancer detection using MR imaging. In addition, it is noteworthy that current risk-based screening recommendations only rely on known risk factors, and that most women with breast cancer have no known risk factors before diagnosis. For example, 89% of women with breast cancer do not have a first-degree family history, and 90% to 95% of these women have no known genetic mutations.[80,81] It is thus likely that there are women with underestimated risk. As previously discussed, supplemental

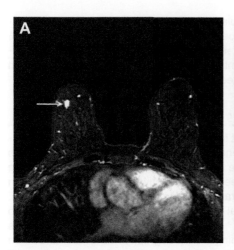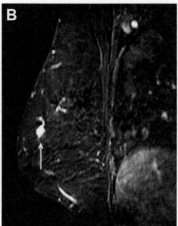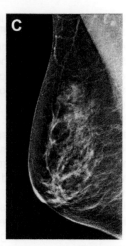

Fig. 3. A 61-year-old woman with *BRCA2* mutation and heterogeneously dense breast tissue with an MR imaging–detected small HER2+ invasive breast cancer in the right breast, as shown in axial (*A*) and sagittal (*B*) projections of postcontrast T1-weighted (T1W) subtraction images (*arrows*). This small invasive ductal carcinoma was identified on supplemental screening MR imaging following negative screening mammogram (*C*) and ultrasonography 5 months prior, and did not have axillary nodal spread at the time of diagnosis.

MR imaging has been shown to be of value, for example, in the subpopulation with dense breast tissue.

MAGNETIC RESONANCE IMAGING SCREENING OUTCOMES
Multimodality Comparison

MR imaging screening has focused on women at high risk for breast cancer; therefore, screening outcomes using MR imaging are primarily based on the high-risk population, which in itself has a higher disease prevalence and lower mammographic sensitivity. Compared with mammography and sonography, MR imaging has a significantly higher sensitivity for all breast cancers. The average sensitivity of MR imaging is around 95%, compared with 40% for mammography and 45% for ultrasonography based on prospective trial data, with MR imaging yielding an additional 8 to 13 per 1000 cancers not otherwise detected by mammography and/or sonography (see **Table 1**).[3,4,11–13,22,23,66] Additional cancer yield is greatest at prevalent round MR imaging screening and decreases at subsequent incident rounds of screening, because of initial capture of cancers that had gone undetected by routine mammography or sonography.[4,12,13,22,66] MR imaging sensitivity particularly outshines that of mammography for small node-negative invasive cancers[7,12,66,82](Fig. 3). For example, in a large randomized trial published in the Lancet in 2019 evaluating 4 rounds of screening in 1355 women, MR imaging not only detected more cancers than mammography (40 vs 15 cancers;

$P = .0017$) but also detected smaller and less frequently node-positive cancers (median size, 9 mm vs 17 mm; $P = .010$) (11% vs 63%; $P = .014$), resulting in a significant shift in tumor stage in the MR imaging group and suggesting a potential for improved survival.[12] Furthermore, a divergent trend of MR imaging preferentially detecting invasive and higher-grade in situ disease as opposed to mammography preferentially detecting in situ and lower-grade invasive disease has been observed,[77] highlighting inherent differences between functional and anatomic depiction of breast cancer. Although direct assessment of MR imaging–specific effect on long-term breast cancer survival is not available, there are consistent data showing significant improvement of at least near-term survival (10-year survival) in high-risk women who undergo MR imaging screening compared with those who do not, because of early detection of more aggressive disease.[7,12] In addition, supplemental MR imaging screening in addition to mammography over multiple rounds has also been observed to curtail interval cancer rates by up to 50%, capturing tumors with worse prognostic features and poorer survival outcomes, and is therefore expected to improve mortality.[12,68,76]

False-Positives

The specificity of breast MR imaging is moderate and typically less than that of mammography in early studies (wide-ranging specificities, 56%–98%[23,82]); however, it has improved over time as imaging technique and clinical experience have matured (higher specificities, often >95% [95%–

98%], reported in recent studies[1–4]). In particular, there is a consistent and significant improvement of specificity from the prevalent round to the incident rounds of screening in prospective trials across multiple years (range, 82%–85% vs 92%–96%), suggesting that limited specificity may be less problematic in the setting of ongoing MR imaging screening.[13,22] The positive predictive value (PPV$_3$) of MR imaging biopsy currently ranges between 20% and 56%, which is comparable with that of mammography (26%–71%), with MR imaging biopsy positivity overrepresented by invasive rather than in situ malignancy (see **Table 1**).[3,4,11–13,22,23,66] In addition, a recent study from 2018 evaluating false-positive findings at multimodality screening found that MR imaging lesions that underwent biopsy were twice as likely to contain atypia than mammographic or tomographic lesions at biopsy, which potentially has implications in risk-based screening regimens.[83] Compared with supplemental MR imaging screening, which yields an additional 10 to 15 per 1000 cancers compared with mammography with a small loss in specificity, supplemental ultrasonography yields only 3 to 4 per 1000 additional cancers with further loss in specificity without improvement in sensitivity compared with MR imaging. For example, in a prospective multimodality trial involving 2662 patients, the number of screens needed to detect 1 cancer was 127 for mammography, 234 for supplemental ultrasonography, and 68 for MR imaging following negative mammogram and ultrasonography examinations.[66]

False-Negatives

MR imaging does not detect all breast cancers. Particularly in the high-risk population, most prospective studies show nonzero interval cancer rates despite annual supplemental MR imaging screening using modern technology (magnets and dedicated breast coils of 1.5–3 T), because of a highly aggressive subset of breast cancers that are rapidly growing, outpacing the frequency of screening[11–13] (see **Table 1**). In contrast, low-grade ductal carcinoma in situ, which typically manifests as microcalcifications best seen on mammography and may not enhance on MR imaging, contributes to most of a small incremental MR imaging–occult cancer yield at mammography (0%–12.5%).[12,13,22,23] The relevance of these false-negative findings on MR imaging is unknown but questionable, given unlikely mortality significance and current debate of overdiagnosis and overtreatment with regard to in situ disease. Retrospective data suggest that concurrent mammography may be of little value in younger high-risk

women undergoing MR imaging screening (age<50 years), who may benefit from reduced radiation dose by forgoing mammography.[84,85] Furthermore, the limited incremental yield of mammography compared with MR imaging is also unlikely to improve despite technological advancement of DBT. For example, in a recent review of 4418 screening MR imaging scans performed either following a negative DBT or a negative digital mammography (DM) study, the incremental cancer detection rates did not differ significantly between the 2 groups.[86] In contrast, although ultrasonography provides a higher number of incremental cancers detected in addition to DM (about 3–4 per 1000), it provides little to no incremental yield when MR imaging is performed and may reduce overall specificity by up to 5% to 6%.[13,22,66] Thus, in women who undergo annual MR imaging screening, concurrent mammography primarily provides added sensitivity for in situ disease, and additional ultrasonography has limited value. However, at this time, mammography is recommended by most guidelines as the primary screening test, because it remains the only test with proven long-term mortality benefit.

BARRIERS TO MAGNETIC RESONANCE IMAGING IN SCREENING

Despite the many potential benefits of MR imaging, there are barriers to wider use, primarily caused by limited availability and cost-effectiveness. Dynamic contrast-enhanced (DCE) MR imaging currently has to meet designated technical specifications (in-plane pixel ≤1 mm, slice thickness ≤3 mm), and standard protocols include T2-weighted and T1-weighted precontrast and 3 postcontrast sequences to generate an enhancement kinetic curve. Therefore, typical examination acquisition requires, on average, 20 to 30 minutes per examination. Both long scan time and limited access to MR imaging scanners currently limit wider use of MR imaging. At the patient level, longer examination duration and the need for intravenous contrast are also less tolerated. In addition, the current cost of the examination may be prohibitive. Although MR imaging screening has been found to be cost-effective among very high-risk women, such as *BRCA* mutation carriers, in terms of quality-adjusted life-years gained, it may not be cost-effective in non-*BRCA* high-risk women in its current form, and is less likely to be cost-effective in moderate-risk or average-risk women.[87–89] However, there is evidence to suggest that MR imaging screening has the potential to become more cost-effective than mammography over time if routinely used, particularly if the cost of the examination decreases.[90] Even as MR imaging screening indications continue to evolve, overall adherence to MR imaging among currently eligible women is poor. In 1 study with long-term follow-up, the frequency of MR imaging screening among high-risk women (cancer free with LTR ≥20%) was less than 40%; of the group, 25% at 4 years and 40% at 8 years did not report any form of screening.[91] Therefore, to optimize MR imaging adoption and enable wider use, a significantly streamlined and less costly examination is mandatory. Current efforts therefore focus on shortening the MR imaging examination in order to minimize both examination acquisition time and interpretation time while maintaining high sensitivity. A shorter and better-tolerated examination will reduce the cost by increasing capacity and throughput, thereby improving accessibility. Variations of abbreviated MR imaging protocols have emerged in recent years and early clinical studies have shown promising results, with abbreviated MR imaging usually achieving similar diagnostic accuracy to the full diagnostic MR imaging protocol.[92,93] Ultrafast imaging with high temporal resolution is also being introduced into abbreviated protocols to further enhance performance.[94,95] Details on early outcomes of abbreviated MR imaging are covered in another article in this issue.

Although noncontrast techniques such as diffusion-weighted imaging are also being investigated, such techniques currently have a low sensitivity, particularly for small lesions, compared with contrast-enhanced MR imaging, thus intravenous contrast remains essential at present. Beyond MR imaging, parallel efforts are also underway to investigate other promising functional imaging modalities, such as contrast-enhanced spectral mammography, which has sensitivity comparable with and specificity slightly higher than MR imaging with likely lower costs and better accessibility.[92]

SUMMARY

MR imaging has a clear modality-based advantage compared with mammography and sonography in early breast cancer detection, and its role in screening is evolving. There is strong evidence to support MR imaging screening in high-risk women, and growing interest and varying levels of evidence for MR imaging screening in moderate-risk women. Among those screened with MR imaging, mammography offers a small incremental cancer yield, and ultrasonography is not additive. Although MR imaging screening in the average-risk population has the potential to improve detection of more relevant disease and minimize overdiagnosis, MR imaging in its current form would not be cost-effective. Abbreviated techniques have streamlined MR imaging to improve the feasibility of wider use. However, more robust data are needed to further consolidate and refine the role of MR imaging in breast cancer screening.

CLINICS CARE POINTS

- In women who undergo annual MR imaging for screening, concurrent mammography primarily provides added sensitivity for in-situ disease, but additional sonography has limited value.
- BRCA1 mutation carriers less than 50 years of age who undergo screening have the highest rate of interval cancers despite annual MR imaging and may benefit from increased frequency of screening.
- Unclassified genetic VUS, including BRCA1/2 VUS, without other risk factors are not indications for supplemental screening with MR imaging.

DISCLOSURE

The authors have nothing to disclose pertaining to this work.

REFERENCES

1. Vreemann S, Gubern-Mérida A, Schlooz-Vries MS, et al. Influence of risk category and screening round on the performance of an MR imaging and mammography screening program in carriers of the BRCA mutation and other women at increased risk. Radiology 2018;286(2):443–51.
2. Kuhl CK, Strobel K, Bieling H, et al. Supplemental breast MR imaging screening of women with average risk of breast cancer. Radiology 2017; 283(2):361–70.
3. Sardanelli F, Podo F, Santoro F, et al. Multicenter surveillance of women at high genetic breast cancer risk using mammography, ultrasonography, and contrast-enhanced magnetic resonance imaging (the High Breast Cancer Risk Italian 1 Study): Final results. Invest Radiol 2011;(46):94–105.
4. Kuhl C, Weigel S, Schrading S, et al. Prospective multicenter cohort study to refine management recommendations for women at elevated familial risk of breast cancer: the EVA trial. J Clin Oncol 2010; 28(9):1450–7.
5. Mann RM, Nariya C, Moy L. Breast MRI: state of the art. Radiology 2019;293(3):520–36.

6. Warner E, Kimberley H, Causer P, et al. Prospective study of breast cancer incidence in women with a BRCA1 or BRCA2 mutation under surveillance with and without magnetic resonance imaging. J Clin Oncol 2011;(29):1664–9.

7. Evans DG, Harkness EF, Howell A, et al. Intensive breast screening in BRCA2 mutation carriers is associated with reduced breast cancer specific and all cause mortality. Heredit Cancer Clin Pract 2016;(14):8.

8. Houssami N. Overdiagnosis of breast cancer in population screening: does it make breast screening worthless? Cancer Biol Med 2017;14(1):1–8.

9. Monticciolo DL, Newell MS, Moy L, et al. Breast cancer screening in women at higher-than-average risk: recommendations from the ACR. J Am Coll Radiol 2018;15(3 Pt A):408–14.

10. Saslow D, Boetes C, Burke W, et al. American Cancer Society guidelines for breast screening with MRI as an adjunct to mammography. CA Cancer J Clin 2007;57(2):75–89.

11. Chiarelli AM, Blackmore KM, Muradali D, et al. Performance measures of magnetic resonance imaging plus mammography in the high risk Ontario Breast Screening Program. J Natl Cancer Inst 2020; 112(2):136–44.

12. Saadatmand S, Amarens Geuzinge H, Rutgers EJT, et al. MRI versus mammography for breast cancer screening in women with familial risk (FaMRIsc): a multicentre, randomised, controlled trial. Lancet Oncol 2019;20(8):1136–47.

13. van Zelst JCM, Mus RDM, Woldringh G, et al. Surveillance of women with the BRCA1 or BRCA2 mutation by using biannual automated breast US, MR imaging, and mammography. Radiology 2017; 285(2):376–88.

14. The American Society of Breast Surgeons - Position statement on screening mammography. 2019. Available at: https://www.breastsurgeons.org/docs/statements/Position-Statement-on-Screening-Mammography.pdf. Accessed May 24, 2020.

15. National Comprehensive Cancer Network (NCCN) Clinical Practice Guidelines in Oncology - Genetic/Familial High-Risk Assessment: Breast, Ovarian, and Pancreatic. Version 1.2020 (Dec. 4, 2019). 2020. Available at: https://www.nccn.org/professionals/physician_gls/pdf/genetics_bop.pdf. Accessed May 21, 2020.

16. National Comprehensive Cancer Network (NCCN) Clinical Practice Guidelines in Oncology – Breast Cancer Screening and Diagnosis. Version 1.2019 (May 17, 2019). 2019. Available at: https://www.nccn.org/professionals/physician_gls/pdf/breast-screening.pdf. Accessed May 21, 2020.

17. Mann RM, Balleyguier C, Baltzer PA, et al. Breast MRI: EUSOBI recommendations for women's information. Eur Radiol 2015;25(12):3669–78.

18. The European Commission Initiative on breast cancer (ECIBC) guidelines for breast cancer screening. Available at: https://healthcare-quality.jrc.ec.europa.eu/european-breast-cancer-guidelines. Accessed April 27, 2020.

19. ACOG (American College of Obstetricians and Gynecologists): Committee on practice bulletins - Gynecology, Committee on genetics, Society of Gynecologic Oncology. Practice Bulletin No 182: Hereditary Breast and Ovarian Cancer Syndrome. Obstet Gynecol 2017;130(3):e110–26.

20. ACOG (American College of Obstetricians and Gynecologists): Committee on Gynecologic Practice. ACOG Committee Opinion no. 593: Management of women with dense breasts diagnosed by mammography. Obstet Gynecol 2014;123(4): 910–1.

21. Antoniou A, Pharoah PDP, Narod S, et al. Average risks of breast and ovarian cancer associated with BRCA1 or BRCA2 mutations detected in case series unselected for family history: A combined analysis of 22 studies. Am J Hum Genet 2003;72(5):1117–30.

22. Riedl CC, Nikolaus L, Bernhart C, et al. Triple-modality screening trial for familial breast cancer underlines the importance of magnetic resonance imaging and questions the role of mammography and ultrasound regardless of patient mutation status, age, and breast density. J Clin Oncol 2015; 33(10):1128–35.

23. Bosse K, Monika G, Gossmann A, et al. Supplemental screening ultrasound increases cancer detection yield in BRCA1 and BRCA2 mutation carriers. Arch Gynecol Obstet 2014;289(3):663–70.

24. Warner E. Screening BRCA1 and BRCA2 mutation carriers for breast cancer. Cancers (Basel) 2018; 10(12):477.

25. Kriege M, Brekelmans CTM, Boetes C, et al. Differences between first and subsequent rounds of the MRISC breast cancer screening program for women with a familial or genetic predisposition. Cancer 2006;106(11):2318–26.

26. Rijnsburger AJ, Inge-Marie O, Kaas R, et al. BRCA1-associated breast cancers present differently from BRCA2-associated and familial cases: Long-term follow-up of Dutch MRISC screening study. J Clin Oncol 2010;28(36):5265–73.

27. Chereau E, Catherine U, Balleyguider C, et al. Characteristics, treatment, and outcome of breast cancers diagnosed in BRCA1 and BRCA2 gene mutation carriers in intensive screening programs including magnetic resonance imaging. Clin Breast Cancer 2010;10(2):113–8.

28. Shah P, Rosen M, Sopfer J, et al. Prospective study of breast MRI in BRCA1 and BRCA2 mutation carriers: effect of mutation status on cancer incidence. Breast Cancer Res Treat 2009;118(3):539–46.

29. Guindalini RSC, Yonglan Z, Abe H, et al. Intensive surveillance with biannual dynamic contrast-enhanced magnetic resonance imaging down-stages breast cancer in BRCA1 mutation carriers. Clin Cancer Res 2019;25(6):1786–94.

30. Plevritis SK, Kurian AW, Sigal BM, et al. Cost-effectiveness of screening BRCA1/2 mutation carriers with breast magnetic resonance imaging. JAMA 2006;295(20):2374–84.

31. Ehsani S, Strigel RM, Pettke E, et al. Screening magnetic resonance imaging recommendations and outcomes in patients at high risk for breast cancer. Breast J 2015;21(3):246–53.

32. Easton DF, Pharoah PDP, Antoniou AC, et al. Gene-panel sequencing and the prediction of breast-cancer risk. N Engl J Med 2015;372(23):2243–57.

33. Shiovitz S, Korde LA. Genetics of breast cancer: a topic in evolution. Ann Oncol 2015;26(7):1291–9.

34. Couch FJ, Hermela S, Hu C, et al. Associations between cancer predisposition testing panel genes and breast cancer. JAMA Oncol 2017;3(9):1190–6.

35. Adank MA, Senno V, Oldenburg RA, et al. Excess breast cancer risk in first degree relatives of CHEK2 *1100delC positive familial breast cancer cases. Eur J Cancer 2013;49(8):1993–9.

36. Antoniou AC, Silvia C, Heikkinen T, et al. Breast-cancer risk in families with mutations in PALB2. N Engl J Med 2014;371(6):497–506.

37. Lakhani SR, Jacquemier J, Sloane JP, et al. Multifactorial analysis of differences between sporadic breast cancers and cancers involving BRCA1 and BRCA2 mutations. J Natl Cancer Inst 1998;90(15): 1138–45.

38. Margolin S, Hemming J, Rutqvist LE, et al. Family history, and impact on clinical presentation and prognosis, in a population-based breast cancer cohort from the Stockholm County. Fam Cancer 2006;2006(5):4.

39. Do WS, Weiss JB, McGregor HF, et al. Poor compliance despite equal access: Military experience with screening breast MRI in high risk women. Am J Surg 2019;217(5):843–7.

40. Beattie MS, Blumenthal E, Creasman J, et al. Abstract P2-02-02: uptake and predictors of screening breast MRI in high risk women. Cancer Res 2010;70(24 supplement). Available at: https://cancerres.aacrjournals.org/content/70/24_Supplement/P2-02-02.

41. Miller JW, Sabatino SA, Thompson TD, et al. Breast MRI use uncommon among U.S. women. Cancer Epidemiol Biomarkers Prev 2013;22(1):159–66.

42. Miles R, Wan F, Onega TL, et al. Underutilization of supplemental magnetic resonance imaging screening among patients at high breast cancer risk. J Womens Health (Larchmt) 2018;27(6): 748–54.

43. The American College of Medical Genetics and Genomics (ACMG) Joint Guidelines for Determining Disease-Causing Potential of DNA Sequence Variations. 2015. Available at: https://www.genome.gov/sites/default/files/media/files/2019-03/American%20College%20of%20Medical%20Genetics%20and%20Genomics%20Report.pdf. Accessed May 23, 2020.

44. Mulder RL, Kremer LCM, Hudson MM, et al. Recommendations for breast cancer surveillance for female survivors of childhood, adolescent, and young adult cancer given chest radiation: a report from the International Late Effects of Childhood Cancer Guideline Harmonization Group. Lancet Oncol 2013;14(13): e621–9.

45. Ehrhardt MJ, Howell CR, Hale K, et al. Subsequent breast cancer in female childhood cancer survivors in the St Jude Lifetime Cohort Study (SJLIFE). J Clin Oncol 2019;37(19):1647–56.

46. Ng AK, Garber JE, Diller LR, et al. Prospective study of the efficacy of breast magnetic resonance imaging and mammographic screening in survivors of Hodgkin lymphoma. J Clin Oncol 2013;31(18): 2282–8.

47. Tieu MT, Cigsar C, Ahmed S, et al. Breast cancer detection among young survivors of pediatric Hodgkin lymphoma with screening magnetic resonance imaging. Cancer 2014;120(16):2507–13.

48. Freitas V, Scaranelo A, Menezes R, et al. Added cancer yield of breast magnetic resonance imaging screening in women with a prior history of chest radiation therapy. Cancer 2013;119(3):495–503.

49. Oeffinger KC, Ford JS, Moskowitz CS, et al. Breast cancer surveillance practices among women previously treated with chest radiation for a childhood cancer. JAMA 2009;301(4):404–14.

50. Nathan PC, Kirsten Kimberlie N, Mahoney MC, et al. Screening and surveillance for second malignant neoplasms in adult survivors of childhood cancer: a report from the childhood cancer survivor study. Ann Intern Med 2010;153(7):442–51.

51. Oeffinger KC, Ford JS, Moskowitz CS, et al. Promoting breast cancer surveillance: The EMPOWER Study, a randomized clinical trial in the Childhood Cancer Survivor Study. J Clin Oncol 2019;37(24): 2131–40.

52. Lee JM, Buist DSM, Houssami N, et al. Five-year risk of interval-invasive second breast cancer. J Natl Cancer Inst 2015;107(7):djv109.

53. Early Breast Cancer Trialists' Collaborative Group (EBCTCG), Darby S, McGale P, et al. Early Breast Cancer Trialists' Collaborative Group (EBCTCG), Effect of radiotherapy after breast-conserving surgery on 10-year recurrence and 15-year breast cancer death: meta-analysis of individual patient data for 10,801 women in 17 randomised trials. Lancet 2011;378(9804):1707–16.

54. Punglia RS, Hassett MJ. Using lifetime risk estimates to recommend magnetic resonance imaging

screening for breast cancer survivors. J Clin Oncol 2010;28(27):4108–10.

55. Mann RM, Kuhl CK, Moy L. Contrast-enhanced MRI for breast cancer screening. J Magn Reson Imaging 2019;50(2):377–90.

56. Wernli KJ, Ichikawa L, Kerlikowske K, et al. Surveillance breast MRI and mammography: Comparison in women with a personal history of breast cancer. Radiology 2019;292(2):311–8.

57. Lehman CD, Lee JM, Demartini WB, et al. Screening MRI in women with a personal history of breast cancer. J Natl Cancer Inst 2016;108(3):djv349.

58. Wanders JO, Holland K, Veldhuis WB, et al. Volumetric breast density affects performance of digital screening mammography. Breast Cancer Res Treat 2017;162(1):5–103.

59. Destounis S, Johnston L, Highnam R, et al. Using volumetric breast density to quantify the potential masking risk of mammographic density. AJR Am J Roentgenol 2017;208(1):222–7.

60. Brandt KR, Scott CG, Ma L, et al. Comparison of clinical and automated breast density measurements: Implications for risk prediction and supplemental screening. Radiology 2016;279(3): 710–9.

61. Boyd NF, Martin LJ, Yaffe MJ, et al. Mammographic density and breast cancer risk: current understanding and future prospects. Breast Cancer Res 2011; 13(6):223.

62. Rafferty EA, Durand MA, Conant EF, et al. Breast cancer screening using tomosynthesis and digital mammography in dense and nondense breasts. JAMA 2016;315:1784–6.

63. Lowry KP, Rebecca Yates C, Miglioretti DL, et al. Screening performance of digital breast tomosynthesis vs digital mammography in community practice by patient age, screening round, and breast density. JAMA Netw Open 2020;3(7):e2011792.

64. Vourtsis A, Berg WA. Breast density implications and supplemental screening. Eur Radiol 2019; 29(4):1762–77.

65. Sprague BL, Stout NK, Schechter C, et al. Benefits, harms, and cost-effectiveness of supplemental ultrasonography screening for women with dense breasts. Ann Intern Med 2015;162(3):157–66.

66. Berg WA, ZZ, Lehrer D, et al. Detection of breast cancer with addition of annual screening ultrasound or a single screening MRI to mammography in women with elevated breast cancer risk. JAMA 2012;307(13):1394–404.

67. FDA (Food and Drug Administration) - Proposed MQSA updates including requirement of breast density reporting. 2019. Available at: https://www. federalregister.gov/documents/2019/03/28/2019-05 803/mammography-quality-standards-act. Accessed May 24, 2020.

68. Bakker MF, de Lange SV, Pijnappel RM, et al. Supplemental MRI screening for women with extremely dense breast tissue. N Engl J Med 2019;381(22): 2091–102.

69. Comstock CE, Gatsonis C, Newstead GM, et al. Comparison of abbreviated breast MRI vs Digital Breast Tomosynthesis for breast cancer detection among women with dense breasts undergoing screening. JAMA 2020;323(8):746–56.

70. King TA, Pilewskie M, Muhsen S, et al. A 29-year longitudinal experience evaluating clinicopathologic features and breast cancer risk. J Clin Oncol 2015; 33(33):3945–52.

71. Page DL, Dupont WD. Premalignant conditions and markers of elevated risk in the breast and their management. Surg Clin North Am 1990;70(4): 831–51.

72. Hartmann LC, Degnim AC, Santen RJ, et al. Atypical hyperplasia of the breast — risk assessment and management options. N Engl J Med 2015;372(1): 78–89.

73. Hartmann LC, Radisky DC, Frost MH, et al. Understanding the premalignant potential of atypical hyperplasia through its natural history: a longitudinal cohort study. Cancer Prev Res (Phila) 2014;7(2): 211–7.

74. Houssami N, Abraham LA, Onega T, et al. Accuracy of screening mammography in women with a history of lobular carcinoma in situ or atypical hyperplasia of the breast. Breast Cancer Res Treat 2014;145(3): 765–73.

75. Burnside ES, Daniel V, Blanks RG, et al. Association between screening mammography recall rate and interval cancers in the UK breast cancer service screening program: A cohort study. Radiology 2018;288(1):47–54.

76. Houssami N, Hunter K. The epidemiology, radiology and biological characteristics of interval breast cancers in population mammography screening. NPJ Breast Cancer 2017;3:12.

77. Sung JS, Sarah S, Brooks J, et al. Breast cancer detected at screening MR imaging and mammography in patients at high risk: method of detection reflects tumor histopathologic results. Radiology 2016; 280(3):716–22.

78. Strigel RM, Jennifer R, Burnside ES, et al. Screening breast MRI outcomes in routine clinical practice: Comparison to BI-RADS benchmarks. Acad Radiol 2017;24(4):411–7.

79. Welch HG, Prorok PC, O'Malley AJ, et al. Breast-cancer tumor size, overdiagnosis, and mammography screening effectiveness. N Engl J Med 2016; 375(15):1438–47.

80. Collaborative Group on Hormonal Factors in Breast Cancer. Familial breast cancer: collaborative reanalysis of individual data from 52 epidemiological studies including 58,209 women with breast cancer

and 101,986 women without the disease. Lancet 2001;358(9291):1389–99.

81. Claus EB, Schildkraut JM, Thompson WD, et al. The genetic attributable risk of breast and ovarian cancer. Cancer 1996;77(11):2318–24.

82. Warner E, Messersmith H, Causer P, et al. Systematic review: using magnetic resonance imaging to screen women at high risk for breast cancer. Ann Intern Med 2008;148(9):671–9.

83. Kuhl CK, Annika K, Strobel K, et al. Not all false positive diagnoses are equal: On the prognostic implications of false-positive diagnoses made in breast MRI versus in mammography/digital tomosynthesis screening. Breast Cancer Res 2018;20(1):13.

84. Vreemann S, van Zelst JCM, Schlooz-Vries M, et al. The added value of mammography in different age-groups of women with and without BRCA mutation screened with breast MRI. Breast Cancer Res 2018;20(1):84.

85. Lo G, Scaranelo AM, Aboras H, et al. Evaluation of the utility of screening mammography for high-risk women undergoing screening breast MR imaging. Radiology 2017;285(1):36–43.

86. Roark AA, Dang PA, Niell BL, et al. Performance of screening breast MRI after negative Full-Field Digital Mammography versus after negative Digital Breast Tomosynthesis in women at higher than average risk for breast cancer. AJR Am J Roentgenol 2019;212(2):271–9.

87. Moore SG, PJ Shenoy, Fanucchi L, et al. Cost-effectiveness of MRI compared to mammography for breast cancer screening in a high risk population. BMC Health Serv Res 2009;9:9.

88. Griebsch I, Broem J, Boggis C, et al. Cost-effectiveness of screening with contrast enhanced magnetic resonance imaging vs X-ray mammography of women at a high familial risk of breast cancer. Br J Cancer 2006;95(7):801–10.

89. Pataky R, Armstrong L, Chia S, et al. Cost-effectiveness of MRI for breast cancer screening in BRCA1/2 mutation carriers. BMC Cancer 2013;13:339.

90. Mango VL, Goel A, Mema E, et al. Breast MRI screening for average-risk women: A monte carlo simulation cost-benefit analysis. J Magn Reson Imaging 2019;49(7):e216–21.

91. Schaeffer M, May BJ, Hogan BC, et al. Breast cancer screening adherence at multiple timepoints over eight years among women in a familial cohort. J Clin Oncol 2019;37(15_suppl):1557.

92. Kuhl CK, Simone S, Strobel K, et al. Abbreviated breast magnetic resonance imaging (MRI): first postcontrast subtracted images and maximum-intensity projection-a novel approach to breast cancer screening with MRI. J Clin Oncol 2014;32(22):2304–10.

93. Leithner D, May L, Morris EA, et al. Abbreviated MRI of the breast: Does it provide value? J Magn Reson Imaging 2019;49(7):e85–100.

94. Mann RM, Mus R, van Zelst J, et al. A novel approach to contrast-enhanced breast magnetic resonance imaging for screening: high-resolution ultrafast dynamic imaging. Invest Radiol 2014;49(9):579–85.

95. Abe H, Mori N, Tsuchiya K, et al. Kinetic analysis of benign and malignant breast lesions with ultrafast dynamic contrast-enhanced MRI: Comparison with standard kinetic assessment. AJR Am J Roentgenol 2016;207(5):1159–66.

Abbreviated MR Imaging for Breast Cancer

Laura Heacock, MS, MD*, Alana A. Lewin, MD, Hildegard K. Toth, MD, Linda Moy, MD,
Beatriu Reig, MD, MPH

KEYWORDS

• Breast MR imaging • Abbreviated MR imaging • Breast cancer screening • FAST imaging

KEY POINTS

- Studies have demonstrated that abbreviated breast MR imaging diagnostic accuracy and sensitivity for breast cancer detection is comparable with that of a full diagnostic protocol in screening populations.
- Abbreviated breast MR imaging protocols remain under development, but include, at a minimum, precontrast and postcontrast T1-weighted images.
- Current limitations of abbreviated breast MR imaging include nonscreening applications and the evaluation of invasive lobular carcinomas and low-grade ductal carcinoma in situ.
- Clinical implementation challenges include the current lack of Current Procedural Terminology coding and minimizing turnaround time as well as imaging time.
- Future directions include the implementation of ultrafast and multiparametric protocols.

INTRODUCTION

Breast MR imaging is the most sensitive imaging method for the detection of breast cancer.[1,2] Although mammography remains the gold standard for breast cancer screening,[3–5] numerous high-quality multicenter trials have demonstrated that breast MR imaging detects on average 3 to 4 times as many breast cancers as mammography in patients with a high (>20%–25%) lifetime risk of breast cancer, with cancer detection rates ranging from 14.7 to 16.0 per 1000 women[6–8] (compared with 5.1 per 1000 women in screening mammography).[9] Although traditionally breast MR imaging has been offered as supplemental screening for high-risk women only, increased cancer detection rates with breast MR imaging have been demonstrated in patients with intermediate (15%–20%) lifetime risk[10,11] and even average (<15%) lifetime risk of breast cancer.[12]

Breast MR imaging offers superior cancer detection to screening mammography and ultrasound examination owing to the uptake of gadolinium intravenous contrast and improved tissue contrast. These features of MR imaging allow for the evaluation of real-time, functional wash-in and wash-out of contrast within the breast parenchyma. The increased angiogenesis and vessel permeability in invasive breast cancer[13] results in avid uptake of contrast compared with the background parenchymal enhancement. Early uptake of contrast has also been demonstrated in high-grade ductal carcinoma in situ (DCIS), which may reflect pathologically increased permeability of the ductal membrane in higher grade DCIS owing to protease activity.[14] The physiologic uptake of contrast in high-grade DCIS and invasive cancers explains the increased detection of these more aggressive malignancies on MR imaging when

Department of Radiology, New York University Grossman School of Medicine, 550 First Avenue, New York, NY 10016, USA
* Corresponding author.
E-mail address: Laura.Heacock@nyulangone.org

Radiol Clin N Am 59 (2021) 99–111
https://doi.org/10.1016/j.rcl.2020.09.001

compared with mammography and ultrasound examination.[15]

Despite the clear advantages of breast MR imaging, it is traditionally recommended only to patients who have a high lifetime breast cancer risk.[2] Recent guidelines have suggested a benefit for women an intermediate lifetime risk as well.[11] Despite these recommendations, only 1.5% of women with a high lifetime risk in the community have ever had a breast MR imaging.[16] This low use likely primarily reflects the traditional high cost of this examination, with cost-effectiveness studies previously showing maximum usefulness in high-risk patients. Other factors often cited in the low use of breast MR imaging include patient tolerance, accessibility, and patient claustrophobia.[17,18]

Abbreviated breast MR imaging, in which a limited number of breast imaging sequences are obtained, has been proposed as a way to solve both cost and patient tolerance issues while preserving the high cancer detection rate of breast MR imaging. Numerous studies have shown that abbreviated breast MR imaging screening can considerably decrease table time and reading time compared with a full breast MR imaging, while offering the same high positive predictive value and diagnostic accuracy.[19–22] The recent Eastern Cooperative Oncology Group-American College of Radiology Imaging Network EA1141 multicenter trial has offered the first proof of the increased cancer detection rate of abbreviated breast MR imaging in average risk patients compared with digital breast tomosynthesis (DBT),[19] paving the way for wider adoption of this screening method.

The purpose of this review is to discuss (1) the background of abbreviated MR imaging, (2) the various proposed abbreviated MR imaging protocols, (3) the known limitations of the modality, and (4) the challenges of clinical implementation.

IMAGING TECHNIQUE

Abbreviated breast MR imaging was first described by Kuhl and colleagues[21] in 2014. In this landmark work, Kuhl and colleagues evaluated 443 women with average to intermediate lifetime risk in a series of 606 screening MR imaging and demonstrated that the diagnostic accuracy and positive predictive value were equivalent between an abbreviated protocol and a full breast imaging protocol. Kuhl's protocol included a noncontrast T1-weighted and a single postcontrast T1-weighted sequence, with generated subtraction images (first postcontrast acquisition subtracted [FAST]) and maximum intensity projection (MIP) images. The average imaging time was 3 minutes compared with a full protocol time of 17 minutes table time; interpretation time was 28 seconds for the FAST images. Although Kuhl's protocol consists of the stripped-down essentials for an abbreviated protocol, multiple iterations have been subsequently proposed (Table 1).

This initial abbreviated protocol can be compared with the American College of Radiology accreditation requirements for breast MR imaging, which include a scout localizer, T2-weighted images and precontrast and postcontrast T1-weighted images.[23] Postcontrast images must include both early and delayed images; generally, at least 3 postcontrast series are acquired. Postprocessing often includes subtraction and MIP images. Additional specialized sequences may include diffusion weighted imaging (DWI), ultrafast (<10 second temporal resolution), and other multiparametric imaging sequences.[10] For this full MR protocol, average table time is approximately 17 to 35 minutes, and this is generally scheduled in a 30- to 60-minute time slot (Fig. 1).

SCREENING PROTOCOL LITERATURE
Overview

Since Kuhl and colleagues first evaluated abbreviated breast MR imaging, more than 5600 examinations in more than 8 countries have been evaluated in retrospective or prospective research studies, including a wide variety of patient populations including patients with average, intermediate, and high lifetime risks of breast cancer.[20,24–29] Despite the heterogeneity of the protocols and patient populations, abbreviated breast MR imaging has consistently demonstrated excellent reproducibility with similar accuracy and sensitivity seen across these studies (see Table 1). These findings suggest that abbreviated breast MR imaging has the potential to increase breast MR imaging screening use by offering a less expensive, shorter examination that is well-tolerated by patients while preserving the high sensitivity of breast MR imaging for biologically aggressive breast cancer.[15] Various sequences can be included in an abbreviated breast MR imaging protocol; the literature to date has explored the usefulness of which sequences should be included in this examination.

Use of Maximum Intensity Projection Images

Early studies of abbreviated MR imaging first determined the minimum number of images that needed to be included in a screening protocol. Kuhl and colleagues evaluated the diagnostic accuracy of MIP images alone compared with FAST images and the full diagnostic protocol,

Table 1
Summary of sequences included in various abbreviated MR imaging protocols and the reported sensitivity, specificity and area under the curve for that protocol

Reference	Ultrafast	Standard Temporal Resolution Pre- T1W	FAST T1W	Second/ Delayed Post T1W	T2W	Sub	MIP	Sens	Spec	Max Area Under the Curve
Platel et al,[61] 2014	Y	Y	Y	N	N	Y	Y	NA	NA	0.87
Kuhl et al,[21] 2014	N	Y	Y	N	N	Y	Y	100%	94.3%	NA
Mann et al,[28] 2014	Y	N	N	N	N	N	N	90%	67%	0.812
Mango et al,[22] 2015	N	Y	Y	N	N	Y	Y	93%–98%	NA	NA
Grimm et al,[32] 2015	N	Y	Y	Y	Y	Y	N	86%–89%	45%–52%	NA
Harvey et al,[20] 2016	N	Y	Y	N	N	Y	Y	100%	94%	NA
Heacock et al,[26] 2016	N	Y	Y	N	Y	Y	N	97.8%–99.4%	NA	NA
Moschetta et al,[33] 2016	N	Y	Y	N	Y	Y	Y	89%	91%	NA
Abe et al,[39] 2016	Y	Y	Y	N	N	Y	N	85%	79%	0.89
Machida et al,[27] 2017	Y	Y	Y	N	N	N	N	87.1%–93.5%	83.4%–91.7%	NA
Chen et al,[24] 2017	N	Y	Y	N	N	Y	Y	92.9%–93.8%	86.5%–88.3%	NA
Petrillo et al,[62] 2017	N	Y	Y	N	N	Y	Y	99.5%	75.4%	NA
Panigrahi et al,[29] 2017	N	Y	Y	N	N	Y	Y	81.8%	97.2%	NA
Romeo et al,[63] 2017	N	Y	Y	N	Y	Y	N	99%	93%	NA
Oldrini et al,[38] 2017	Y	Y	Y	N	Y	Y	N	93.1%	70.8%–83.3%	NA
Choi et al,[25] 2017	N	Y	Y	N	Y	Y	Y	100%	89.2%	NA
Oldrini et al,[64] 2018	N	Y	Y	N	N	Y	N	100%	95.1%	NA
Lee-Felker et al,[65] 2019	N	Y	Y	N	N	Y	Y	99%	97%	NA

Studies that used an ultrafast sequence had a temporal resolution of less than 10 s and were run both before and after contrast injection.

Abbreviations: FAST, first post contrast; Max, maximum; N, no; Pre, precontrast; Sens, sensitivity; Spec, specificity; Subs, subtraction images; T1W, T1-weighted; T2W, T2-weighted; Y, yes.

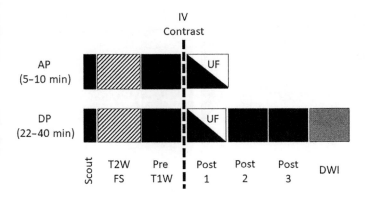

Fig. 1. Comparison of a typical abbreviated breast MR imaging protocol (AP) with a typical diagnostic breast MR imaging protocol (DP). At a minimum, the AP should include precontrast and first postcontrast T1-weighted images, with generated subtraction images and MIP image if desired. T2-weighted images are required for ACR MR imaging accreditation requirements. Ultrafast imaging and diffusion weighted imaging can be included in either AP or DP as part of a multiparametric protocol. FS, fat saturated; Post 1, first postcontrast T1-weighted; Pre T1W, precontrast T1-weighted; T2W, T2 weighted; UF, ultrafast.

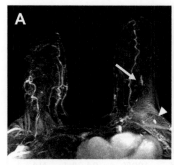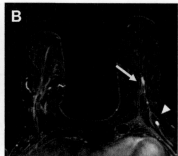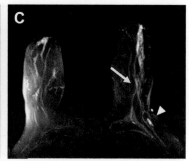

Fig. 2. A 73-year-old woman with a strong family history of breast cancer. MR imaging performed for intermediate-risk screening. In the left breast at 3:00 there is a 1.0-cm linear nonmass enhancement (*arrow*), seen on both MIP image (*A*) and corresponding first postcontrast subtraction images (*B*). There is no correlate on T2-weighted images (*C*). MR imaging guided biopsy yielded high-grade DCIS. The *arrowhead* denotes an incidental, stable, intramammary lymph node with corresponding increased T2-weighted signal.

with 11 cancers evaluated in 606 screening MR imaging examinations. Although MIP interpretation time was substantially shorter at 2.8 seconds, 10 of 11 cancers were identified. FAST image interpretation was 28 seconds and all 11 cancers were seen, equivalent to the full diagnostic protocol (Fig. 2). The specificity and positive predictive value were also equivalent between FAST images and full diagnostic protocol (94.3% vs 93.9% and 24.4% vs 23.4%, respectively; *P* = .563[21]). Kuhl and colleagues concluded that FAST image interpretation may be preferable to MIP alone. This finding was reinforced by Mango and colleagues,[22] who evaluated 100 biopsy-proven unicentric breast cancers in a 4-reader study using the same sequences as Kuhl and associates. The first postcontrast subtraction image interpretation had a sensitivity of 96% compared with 93% for MIP images. Abbreviated MR imaging acquisition time was 10 to 15 minutes compared with a full protocol of 30 to 40 minutes, with an average interpretation time of 44 seconds (Fig. 3). In this study evaluating only known

cancers, missed lesions were more likely to be low-grade invasive cancer or DCIS. Although MIP evaluation can be useful for a quick overview, FAST images should be reviewed carefully to detect subtle lesions.

Usefulness of Additional Postcontrast Sequences

The most commonly described abbreviated MR protocol includes only a single early postcontrast sequence, and there are few studies of later postcontrast sequences. In the American College of Radiology Breast Imaging and Reporting Data System lexicon, enhancement of breast lesions is broken into the initial phase, which represents peak enhancement in the first 2 minutes, and the delayed phase, which occurs after 2 minutes.[30] The signal intensity over time creates a time intensity curve, which may show persistent, plateau, or washout enhancement. The time–intensity curves are known to be differently distributed among malignant and benign lesions, with significant

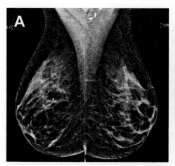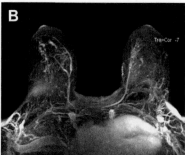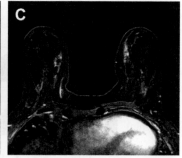

Fig. 3. A 45-year-old woman with a strong family history of breast cancer presenting for high-risk screening. Annual mammogram demonstrates heterogeneously dense breasts (*A*). MIP image (*B*) and corresponding first postcontrast image (*C*) are negative. Compared with routine diagnostic breast MR imaging, abbreviated breast MR imaging interpretation time has been reported as less than 2 minutes on average.

overlap.[31] In adding additional postcontrast sequences to the abbreviated protocol, investigators seek to capture some of the kinetic information that is available in the full MR imaging protocol.

A reader study of 48 high-risk screening MR imaging studies comparing a full protocol with abbreviated protocols with only the first postcontrast sequence versus with the addition of the second postcontrast sequence found no significant difference in sensitivity and specificity between the protocols.[32] In fact, the addition of the second postcontrast sequence resulted in a nonsignificant trend toward a lower specificity compared with the first postcontrast sequence only. In this study, scan time for each sequence was 2 minutes, such that the second postcontrast sequence was in the early delayed phase (or intermediate phase).

Seeking to capture information from the intermediate phase of the postcontrast period, Moschetta and colleagues[33] evaluated an abbreviated protocol using a more delayed single postcontrast sequence obtained 3 minutes after injection. In comparison with the full dynamic contrast-enhanced MR imaging, there was no difference in sensitivity, specificity, or accuracy. The authors argue that, rather than attempt to evaluate dynamic enhancement over time, their protocol preferentially evaluated the presence of enhancement and the morphology of lesions on high-resolution postcontrast images. However, note that the authors did not compare their abbreviated protocol with this delayed sequence with a more abbreviated protocol using only an earlier postcontrast sequence.

Choudhery and colleagues[34] compared full dynamic contrast-enhanced MR imaging with an abbreviated MR imaging protocol composed of 2 postcontrast sequences. These sequences were centered at 60 to 75 seconds and 180 to 205 seconds after injection and the investigators generated time–intensity curves. They found no significant differences in the time–intensity curve types of benign versus malignant lesions as obtained with either the full or abbreviated protocol. Malignant lesions seen on the abbreviated protocol demonstrated persistent time–intensity curve in 60.7% of lesions, plateau curve in 24.6%, and washout in 14.8%, which was not significantly different from the full protocol. However, with the full protocol, there was a nonsignificant trend toward more washout and fewer plateau curves in malignant lesions as compared with the abbreviated protocol, similar to the findings of Partridge and colleagues.[35] Note that this was not a reader study and the clinical usefulness of the time–intensity curves was not assessed. However, this study demonstrated significant overlap between worst curve types seen in benign and malignant lesions, suggesting kinetic information may not have improved lesion characterization.

Park and colleagues[36] compared screening women with a personal history of breast cancer with a full MR imaging protocol versus an abbreviated protocol composed of 2 postcontrast sequences, each of which was 1 minute long. The investigators found the abbreviated MR imaging protocol resulted in decreased sensitivity, increased specificity, and similar accuracy compared with the full MR imaging protocol. In this study, the inclusion of the second sequence was likely important to the sensitivity of the abbreviated examination given that this sequence was timed within the initial phase of lesion enhancement. Therefore, in determining the usefulness of multiple postcontrast sequences, the postcontrast acquisition time of each sequence must be specified given the variability in MR imaging protocols. Overall, adding additional postcontrast sequences beyond the FAST acquisition seems to lengthen imaging time without clinical benefit.

Ultrafast Imaging

An essential premise of abbreviated breast MR imaging is that the first postcontrast images are when cancers are most visible compared with background parenchymal enhancement and that more delayed postcontrast imaging does not increase sensitivity. However, omission of the delayed postcontrast acquisitions also limits kinetic analysis of gadolinium wash-out, which can provide important information for lesion characterization.[31] A proposed substitute is to instead evaluate the wash-in of contrast on abbreviated MR imaging, using new ultrafast and accelerated breast MR imaging techniques. These imaging sequences exploit various k-space undersampling and view-sharing techniques to continuously sample the center of k-space while sparsely sampling peripheral regions of k-space over time, allowing for temporal resolution of 10 frames per second or less with relative preservation of spatial resolution.[28,37,38] Ultrafast sequences can therefore image the wash-in of contrast every 1 to 10 seconds during the first 1 to 2 minutes postcontrast, compared with a standard temporal resolution of 2 to 3 minutes in routine diagnostic breast MR imaging. This protocol allows for early visualization of angiogenic lesions with minimization of background parenchymal enhancement (**Fig. 4**).

Investigation of early contrast wash-in as measured by ultrafast techniques has demonstrated important differences between malignant and benign lesions. One such ultrafast abbreviated

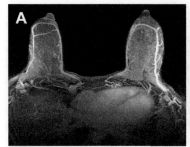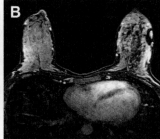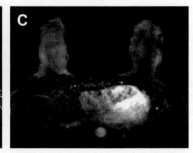

Fig. 4. A 42-year-old woman with BRCA1 mutation presenting for high-risk screening while breastfeeding. MIP images (*A*) and first postcontrast T1-weighted images (*B*) demonstrate diffuse marked background parenchymal enhancement consistent with lactational changes and limiting sensitivity for breast cancer detection. However, ultrafast time-resolved angiography with interleaved stochastic trajectories images with 4-second temporal resolution after contrast injection performed on a 3.0T magnet (*C*) demonstrate no early wash-in of contrast in either breast at 12-second postcontrast injection, consistent with a negative study. Use of ultrafast imaging to evaluate early wash-in of contrast allows for evaluation of the breasts at optimal timing to minimize background parenchymal enhancement. In this abbreviated protocol, ultrafast imaging is performed with a slightly decreased spatial resolution and then followed by a high spatial resolution volumetric interpolated breath-hold examination sequence to allow for lesion characterization.

breast MR imaging protocol by Mann and colleagues[28] used time-resolved angiography with interleaved stochastic trajectories imaging to evaluate 160 patients, with maximum slope of contrast wash-in demonstrating higher area under the curve (0.829) than standard Breast Imaging and Reporting Data System criteria (AUC, 0.692). In addition to maximum slope, enhancement ratios also differ between benign and malignant lesions; Abe and colleagues[39] evaluated the initial enhancement rate and signal enhancement ratio in 62 lesions and found increased initial enhancement rate and signal enhancement ratio correlated with malignancy. Although ultrafast kinetic information remains experimental, it seems to offer valuable supplemental information similar to the role of kinetic curve wash-out information in full diagnostic breast MR imaging.

T2-Weighted Imaging

Although T1-weighted precontrast and postcontrast images are the mainstay of abbreviated breast MR imaging, T2-weighted images are considered a minimal requirement for American College of Radiology breast MR imaging recommendation[23] and are often included in abbreviated MR imaging protocols. In early studies of diagnostic breast MR imaging, T2-weighted images were shown to improve lesion characterization and showed[40,41] usefulness in distinguishing benign from malignant lesions. More recent studies evaluating modern breast MR imaging have shown mixed usefulness.[10] However, a perceived drawback of abbreviated MR imaging is that it may result in more short-term follow-up

studies than full diagnostic breast MR imaging.[21,42] As such, inclusion of T2-weighted imaging may be of interest in future studies to decrease Breast Imaging and Reporting Data System 3 recommendations and decrease unnecessary short-term follow-up (**Fig. 5**).

Heacock and colleagues[26] found the addition of T2-weighted imaging did not change cancer detection rate in a series of 107 known unilateral breast cancers. However, all 3 readers reported that reviewing the T2-weighted images increased lesion conspicuity. Adding T2-weighted images increased scan time to 5 minutes, but only increased reader interpretation time by 5 to 10 seconds. The authors noted that, because the study was performed in a population of known breast cancers, the usefulness of T2-weighted imaging may be limited in changing diagnostic accuracy; T2-weighted imaging is likely most helpful in the screening setting. In a subsequent study, Strahle and colleagues[43] evaluated various protocol combinations in evaluating 452 mixed benign and malignant lesions. Statistical analysis demonstrated that the most effective sequence order and inclusion was T2-weighted images, T1-weighted precontrast, and T1-weighted first and late postcontrast breast MR imaging had the greatest sensitivity and specificity in breast cancer screening. The total scan time for this protocol was 7.5 minutes.

Although abbreviated MR imaging both with and without T2-weighted imaging demonstrate similar accuracy, many early studies were not performed in pure screening populations. Numerous studies have subsequently included T2-weighted imaging

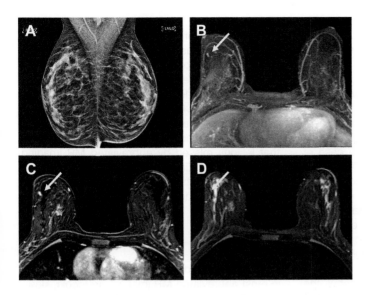

Fig. 5. A 32-year-old BRCA-positive woman presenting for high-risk screening. A mammogram performed 6 months earlier (A) demonstrates heterogeneously dense breasts with no mammographic abnormality. An oval circumscribed mass (arrow) in the right breast at 10:00 anterior depth is seen on MIP image (B) and first postcontrast subtraction images (C) with no correlate on T2-weighted images (D). Although the addition of T2-weighted sequences has not been demonstrated to increase cancer detection rates, it improves reader confidence in diagnosis and may decrease short-term follow-up recommendations in the screening setting. MR imaging-guided biopsy found invasive ductal carcinoma.

without specifically evaluating the impact of this sequence, including the recent Eastern Cooperative Oncology Group-American College of Radiology Imaging Network 1141 multicenter trial. Standardized MR imaging interpretation in EA1141 specifically includes the presence or absence of T2-weighted imaging in determining whether or not to biopsy or follow an enhancing lesion on screening MR imaging.[19] It remains undetermined if the inclusion of T2-weighted imaging changes breast cancer detection, but similar to full diagnostic imaging, it likely is most valuable in increasing specificity and biopsy positive predictive value.

Noncontrast, Diffusion-Weighted Imaging, and Multiparametric Imaging

With the concerns about safety of gadolinium containing contrast agents and the recommendation that gadolinium-based contrast should only be administered when necessary,[44] noncontrast protocols have been studied with some encouraging results. DWI is a noncontrast MR technique that measures the random motion of water molecules in tissue, reflecting the cellular microenvironment. Studies of noncontrast abbreviated MR protocols with combinations of DWI with T1-weighted and/or T2-weighted sequences yielded sensitivities of 45% to 78% for the detection of malignancy.[45,46] These sensitivities are at least similar to[46] or higher than mammography,[45] but do not compare favorably with the higher sensitivity for cancer detection of contrast-enhanced MR imaging. This finding suggests that DWI may not be ready for use as a stand-alone screening technique. However, DWI

has shown promise in lesion characterization, demonstrating similar accuracy for characterizing benign from malignant lesions as contrast-enhanced MR imaging.[47–49] A study of patients with mammographically detected suspicious lesions used an abbreviated MR imaging protocol of DWI and T2-weighted imaging to characterize the lesions, with a negative predictive value of 0.92 and a positive predictive value of 0.93, which were higher than an abbreviated protocol of the first postcontrast sequence.[47]

The combination of a contrast-enhanced sequence for cancer detection and a DWI sequence for lesion characterization seems to show the most promising results for sensitivity and specificity.[50] A study of screening MR imaging in 356 women found that an abbreviated protocol including DWI had higher sensitivity and specificity than an abbreviated protocol without DWI, with similar sensitivity and specificity as the full protocol.[24] The limitations of DWI have been shown to be in the detection of invasive lobular carcinoma, mucinous cancers, invasive cancers presenting as diffuse nonmass enhancement, and lesions smaller than 12 mm.[50]

EASTERN COOPERATIVE ONCOLOGY GROUP-AMERICAN COLLEGE OF RADIOLOGY IMAGING NETWORK TRIAL RESULTS AND TRIALS IN DEVELOPMENT

The recently published EA1141 trial (Comparison of abbreviated breast MR imaging and DBT in breast cancer screening in women with dense breasts) is a study comparing abbreviated MR imaging against DBT.[19] The investigators enrolled

1510 asymptomatic, average-risk women with dense breasts to undergo both DBT and abbreviated MR imaging screening examinations on the same day. The results of the first round of screening showed that the invasive cancer detection rate of abbreviated MR imaging was more than double that of DBT (11.8 per 1000 compared with 4.8 per 1000). Of the 23 cancers identified, abbreviated MR imaging identified 22 cancers (17 invasive and 4 DCIS) and missed a case of DCIS. DBT identified only 9 cancers (7 invasive and 2 DCIS). Of the 17 total invasive cancers identified in the study, 3 were high grade and all of these were only identified by MR imaging and were missed on DBT. This result is consistent with the prior observation by Sung and colleagues[15] that MR imaging detects higher grade tumors than mammography.

The first-round results of EA1141 show the promise of abbreviated MR imaging as an adjunct screening test in average-risk women. Follow-up is ongoing; patients will undergo a second round of DBT and abbreviated MR imaging screening at the 1-year mark, as an incidence screening round. The EA1141 investigators will also evaluate the types of detected invasive and in situ cancers by genomic profiling, to gain further insight into whether abbreviated MR imaging may identify more biologically aggressive tumors than DBT.

An ongoing large multicenter trial in the United Kingdom, the Breast Screening—Risk Adaptive Imaging for Density (BRAID) trial, will randomize women found to have dense breasts on screening mammography to supplemental screening with either automated breast ultrasound examination, contrast-enhanced spectral mammography, or abbreviated MR imaging (clinicaltrial.gov identifier NCT04097366). There are currently no large trials of abbreviated MR imaging underway in which patients are randomized to be screened with abbreviated MR imaging only, without mammography.

NONSCREENING APPLICATION: EXTENT OF DISEASE EVALUATION

The value of abbreviated MR imaging in the setting of a newly diagnosed cancer has been evaluated by a few small studies. A retrospective reader study of 81 MR imaging studies performed for extent of disease evaluation compared the full protocol MR with an abbreviated MR consisting of precontrast, and first postcontrast T1, MIP, and subtraction sequences.[51] Investigators found no difference between the protocols in detecting multifocal, multicentric, contralateral malignancy, or axillary nodal metastasis. A similar study of 87 patients with known cancer found no difference

between readers' additional lesion detection rate between the full protocol and the abbreviated protocol of precontrast and first postcontrast T1 with MIP image.[52] In both of these studies, out of a total of 9 false-negative lesions missed on abbreviated MR imaging but detected on full protocol MR imaging, all were DCIS and low-grade invasive carcinomas, other than one 5-mm high-grade IDC missed by 1 reader.[52] This outcome suggests that lesions missed by abbreviated MR imaging may not be as clinically relevant in patients who will be treated with locoregional radiation and systemic therapy. Additional research in this area is needed.

LIMITATIONS

Given the lack of delayed postcontrast sequences in most abbreviated MR imaging protocols, slow-enhancing malignancies may be missed. These neoplasms include invasive lobular carcinoma, DCIS, and invasive ductal carcinoma presenting as nonmass enhancement.[22,26]

In addition, residual invasive or in situ cancer after neoadjuvant therapy may be missed. Neoadjuvant chemotherapy or endocrine therapy, which is administered before breast surgery, may be used in selected patients to shrink tumor size in the breast and axilla. Post-treatment MR imaging is the most sensitive modality to evaluate extent of residual disease and enable accurate surgical planning.[53] The antiangiogenic effects of chemotherapy may result in delayed enhancement of residual invasive disease.[54] Residual DCIS may also demonstrate delayed enhancement[55] and its extent is important to delineate to achieve negative surgical margins and avoid re-excision. For these reasons, the use of abbreviated MR in post-treatment imaging may not be successful and has not been prospectively studied.[10]

For abbreviated MR imaging protocols that rely on evaluation of the MIP image, lesions at the periphery of the field of view may be missed, such as those in the axilla[22,26] and chest wall[32] (Fig. 6).

CLINICAL IMPLEMENTATION

Research to date has demonstrated that abbreviated breast MR imaging has promise in increasing the use of screening MR imaging. Radiologists are increasingly expected to demonstrate the quality and appropriateness of advanced imaging techniques such as breast MR imaging, particularly as reimbursement and health care policy shift from a fee-for-service model to value-based health care.[56] To gain widespread acceptance for supplemental screening, abbreviated breast MR

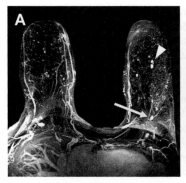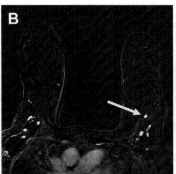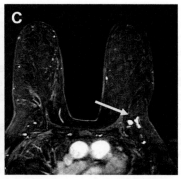

Fig. 6. A 56-year-old woman with a personal history of atypia and a strong family history of breast cancer, presenting for high-risk screening. An oval, homogenously enhancing 0.8-cm mass in the left breast at 2:00 (*arrow*) seems to be a benign axillary lymph node on MIP image (*A*), but is slightly anterior to axillary lymph nodes on corresponding first postcontrast subtraction images (*B*). However, the mass is new compared with prior MR imaging (*C*). MR imaging-guided biopsy yielded metaplastic carcinoma. *Arrowhead* denotes a previously biopsied left breast benign masses. Axillary lesions are a known pitfall of MIP interpretation; this area should be reviewed carefully on first postcontrast images.

imaging will need to demonstrate that it decreases costs while improving patient outcomes. One ongoing secondary analysis of the recently completed EA1141 study is a cost-effectiveness analysis comparing abbreviated MR imaging with DBT.[19] It is anticipated that the projected lower cost of this examination combined with its high diagnostic accuracy will result in favorable cost-effectiveness analysis compared with a standard breast MR imaging. Practices seeking to offer abbreviated breast MR imaging in the meantime have important reimbursement and workflow considerations that must be addressed.

Reimbursement

There is currently no Current Procedural Terminology code for abbreviated MR imaging and thus most imaging facilities offering abbreviated breast MR imaging inform patients up front that the study is self-pay and not covered by insurance. Although individual facilities have various inclusion criteria, abbreviated breast MR imaging is often offered to patients at average risk with dense breasts or patients with intermediate lifetime risk as a supplemental screening examination,[42] because these women may not meet insurance coverage requirements for MR imaging screening (reserved for high-risk women) and thus have higher out-of-pocket costs. In contrast, patients who have a high lifetime risk of breast cancer usually have routine insurance coverage for breast MR imaging and can undergo the standard diagnostic examination. If a high-risk patient has a high-deductible health insurance plan, however, the patient may also prefer the up-front cost of the abbreviated MR imaging to that of their deductible

for the full examination. Considerations when establishing the cost of the examination can include regional pricing for other breast screening examinations and similar screening examinations, such as unhenanced lung cancer computed tomography scans and cardiac calcium scoring.[42] In limited states, such as Michigan, abbreviated breast MR imaging is covered by health maintenance organizations.

Clinical Workflow

Clinical workflow implementation remains a key consideration in offering abbreviated breast MR imaging. Of note, the majority of research studies evaluate abbreviated MR imaging time or scan time, which is not equivalent with "table time" or the complete time it takes to evaluate a patient. This time includes preparing the patient for the examination, the scan time, and the time to turn around the room for the next patient. Borthakur and colleagues[57] evaluated scan time and complete study time between abbreviated breast MR imaging and full breast MR imaging screening studies and found that scan time for their abbreviated protocol was 17.5 minutes with a total study time of 36 minutes; this compared with scan time of 28.8 minutes for the full protocol and total study time of 50 minutes. When comparing total study time, the abbreviated protocol had only a 38% greater patient flow rate than the standard breast MR imaging despite a 65% decrease in scan time, with increased technologist activity time explaining the discrepancy between scan and study time savings.[57] This finding emphasizes that workflow must be optimized to maximize efficiency when implementing abbreviated breast MR imaging, because this information is critical to estimating the price point for an abbreviated study and assessing feasibility for widespread implementation.

A critical look at current and projected workflow for breast MR imaging is therefore important to adding value when implementing an abbreviated protocol. One easy to implement solution is to batch schedule abbreviated breast MR imaging patients in consecutive slots, as suggested by Marshall and colleagues.[42] Imaging abbreviated breast MR imaging patients consecutively allows for the technologist workstation setup and breast coil to remain in place, maximizing patient turnaround efficiency. A more challenging solution to implement is to critically evaluate general MR imaging workflow. Space and funds permitting, dockable tables, duplication of coils, and optimizing the patient's path to the scanner can result in time savings even when scanning a heterogeneous set of daily protocols.[58] Finally, workflow considerations need also include radiologist interpretation time. Although reported abbreviated breast MR imaging interpretation time is generally reported to be less than 5 minutes in the research setting,[21] this time does not include a review of patient history and prior examinations, both of which can be expected to increase interpretation time.

FUTURE DIRECTIONS

Although it is clear that abbreviated breast MR imaging has promise as a screening examination, identifying the populations most likely to benefit from this examination is ongoing. The use of abbreviated breast MR imaging in preoperative breast MR imaging for assessment of breast cancer extent of disease, in problem solving, and in assessment of neoadjuvant chemotherapy response remain underexplored. Other directions of current research involve the incorporation of ultrafast and other multiparametric sequences[10] into abbreviated breast MR imaging to increase both its sensitivity and specificity. Another ongoing area of research is the implementation of deep learning techniques, which may be useful both in the interpretation of screening abbreviated MR imaging[59] and in MR imaging reconstruction to provide additional information and further decrease scan time.[60]

SUMMARY

MR imaging is the most sensitive imaging modality for the detection of breast cancer, far outperforming full-field digital mammography, tomosynthesis, and ultrasound examination. However, the long examination time of breast MR imaging increases the cost and decreases examination availability, making it impractical as a large-scale screening examination. Abbreviated MR imaging has been shown to have similar diagnostic accuracy as full protocol MR imaging, with significantly shortened examination time. Further studies are still needed to standardize the abbreviated protocol, to refine the patient population most likely to benefit from abbreviated MR imaging, and to evaluate outcomes in patients with abbreviated MR imaging -detected cancers.

CLINICS CARE POINTS

- Abbreviated breast MR imaging has diagnostic accuracy and sensitivity for breast cancer detection comparable to that of a full diagnostic protocol in screening populations
- Minimal protocol requirements for abbreviated breast MR imaging include precontrast and postcontrast T1-weighted images. T2-weighted imaging may be necessary to meet American College of Radiology breast MR imaging accreditation requirements.
- The use of abbreviated breast MR imaging in nonscreening applications (eg, known breast cancer extent of disease evaluation, problem solving, and postneoadjuvant chemotherapy evaluation) remains under investigation.
- Clinical challenges to implementation include reimbursement considerations and optimization of workflow to maximize patient turnaround.

DISCLOSURE

The authors state no relevant conflict of interest or financial disclosures.

REFERENCES

1. Sardanelli F, Boetes C, Borisch B, et al. Magnetic resonance imaging of the breast: recommendations from the EUSOMA working group. Eur J Cancer 2010;46(8):1296–316.
2. Saslow D, Boetes C, Burke W, et al. American Cancer Society guidelines for breast screening with MRI as an adjunct to mammography. CA Cancer J Clin 2007;57(2):75–89.
3. Monticciolo DL, Newell MS, Hendrick RE, et al. Breast Cancer Screening for Average-Risk Women: recommendations From the ACR Commission on Breast Imaging. J Am Coll Radiol 2017;14(9): 1137–43.
4. Myers ER, Moorman P, Gierisch JM, et al. Benefits and harms of breast cancer screening: a systematic review. JAMA 2015;314(15):1615–34.

5. Sardanelli F, Aase HS, Alvarez M, et al. Position paper on screening for breast cancer by the European Society of Breast Imaging (EUSOBI) and 30 national breast radiology bodies from Austria, Belgium, Bosnia and Herzegovina, Bulgaria, Croatia, Czech Republic, Denmark, Estonia, Finland, France, Germany, Greece, Hungary, Iceland, Ireland, Italy, Israel, Lithuania, Moldova, The Netherlands, Norway, Poland, Portugal, Romania, Serbia, Slovakia, Spain, Sweden, Switzerland and Turkey. Eur Radiol 2017;27(7):2737–43.

6. Berg WA, Zhang Z, Lehrer D, et al. Detection of breast cancer with addition of annual screening ultrasound or a single screening MRI to mammography in women with elevated breast cancer risk. JAMA 2012;307(13):1394–404.

7. Kuhl C, Weigel S, Schrading S, et al. Prospective multicenter cohort study to refine management recommendations for women at elevated familial risk of breast cancer: the EVA trial. J Clin Oncol 2010; 28(9):1450–7.

8. Lehman CD, Isaacs C, Schnall MD, et al. Cancer yield of mammography, MR, and US in high-risk women: prospective multi-institution breast cancer screening study. Radiology 2007;244(2):381–8.

9. Lehman CD, Arao RF, Sprague BL, et al. National performance benchmarks for modern screening digital mammography: update from the breast cancer surveillance consortium. Radiology 2017; 283(1):49–58.

10. Mann RM, Cho N, Moy L. Breast MRI: state of the art. Radiology 2019;292(3):520–36.

11. Monticciolo DL, Newell MS, Moy L, et al. Breast cancer screening in women at higher-than-average risk: recommendations from the ACR. J Am Coll Radiol 2018;15(3 Pt A):408–14.

12. Kuhl CK, Strobel K, Bieling H, et al. Supplemental breast MR imaging screening of women with average risk of breast cancer. Radiology 2017; 283(2):361–70.

13. Buadu LD, Murakami J, Murayama S, et al. Breast lesions: correlation of contrast medium enhancement patterns on MR images with histopathologic findings and tumor angiogenesis. Radiology 1996; 200(3):639–49.

14. Kuhl CK. Why do purely intraductal cancers enhance on breast MR images? Radiology 2009; 253(2):281–3.

15. Sung JS, Stamler S, Brooks J, et al. Breast cancers detected at screening MR imaging and mammography in patients at high risk: method of detection reflects tumor histopathologic results. Radiology 2016; 280(3):716–22.

16. Wernli KJ, DeMartini WB, Ichikawa L, et al. Patterns of breast magnetic resonance imaging use in community practice. JAMA Intern Med 2014;174(1): 125–32.

17. Berg WA, Blume JD, Adams AM, et al. Reasons women at elevated risk of breast cancer refuse breast MR imaging screening: ACRIN 6666. Radiology 2010;254(1):79–87.

18. de Lange SV, Bakker MF, Monninkhof EM, et al. Reasons for (non)participation in supplemental population-based MRI breast screening for women with extremely dense breasts. Clin Radiol 2018; 73(8):759.e1-9.

19. Comstock CE, Gatsonis C, Newstead GM, et al. Comparison of abbreviated breast MRI vs digital breast tomosynthesis for breast cancer detection among women with dense breasts undergoing screening. JAMA 2020;323(8):746–56.

20. Harvey SC, Di Carlo PA, Lee B, et al. An abbreviated protocol for high-risk screening breast MRI saves time and resources. J Am Coll Radiol 2016;13(4): 374–80.

21. Kuhl CK, Schrading S, Strobel K, et al. Abbreviated breast magnetic resonance imaging (MRI): first postcontrast subtracted images and maximum-intensity projection-a novel approach to breast cancer screening with MRI. J Clin Oncol 2014;32(22): 2304–10.

22. Mango VL, Morris EA, David Dershaw D, et al. Abbreviated protocol for breast MRI: are multiple sequences needed for cancer detection? Eur J Radiol 2015;84(1):65–70.

23. ACR. American College of Radiology website. Breast magnetic resonance imaging (MRI) accreditation program requirements 2017. Available at: www.acraccreditation.org/~/media/ACRAccreditation/Documents/Breast-MRI/Requirements.pdf?la=en. Accessed October 17, 2019.

24. Chen SQ, Huang M, Shen YY, et al. Abbreviated MRI Protocols for Detecting Breast Cancer in Women with Dense Breasts. Korean J Radiol 2017;18(3): 470–5.

25. Choi BH, Choi N, Kim MY, et al. Usefulness of abbreviated breast MRI screening for women with a history of breast cancer surgery. Breast Cancer Res Treat 2018;167(2):495–502.

26. Heacock L, Melsaether AN, Heller SL, et al. Evaluation of a known breast cancer using an abbreviated breast MRI protocol: correlation of imaging characteristics and pathology with lesion detection and conspicuity. Eur J Radiol 2016;85(4):815–23.

27. Machida Y, Shimauchi A, Kanemaki Y, et al. Feasibility and potential limitations of abbreviated breast MRI: an observer study using an enriched cohort. Breast Cancer 2017;24(3):411–9.

28. Mann RM, Mus RD, van Zelst J, et al. A novel approach to contrast-enhanced breast magnetic resonance imaging for screening: high-resolution ultrafast dynamic imaging. Invest Radiol 2014;49(9): 579–85.

29. Panigrahi B, Mullen L, Falomo E, et al. An abbreviated protocol for high-risk screening breast magnetic resonance imaging: impact on performance metrics and BI-RADS assessment. Acad Radiol 2017;24(9):1132–8.

30. Morris EA, Comstock CE, Lee CH, et al. ACR BI-RADS® Magnetic Resonance Imaging. In: ACR BI-RADS® Atlas, Breast Imaging Reporting and Data System. Reston (VA): American College of Radiology; 2013.

31. Kuhl CK, Mielcareck P, Klaschik S, et al. Dynamic breast MR imaging: are signal intensity time course data useful for differential diagnosis of enhancing lesions? Radiology 1999;211(1):101–10.

32. Grimm LJ, Soo MS, Yoon S, et al. Abbreviated screening protocol for breast MRI: a feasibility study. Acad Radiol 2015;22(9):1157–62.

33. Moschetta M, Telegrafo M, Rella L, et al. Abbreviated combined MR protocol: a new faster strategy for characterizing breast lesions. Clin Breast Cancer 2016;16(3):207–11.

34. Choudhery S, Chou SS, Chang K, et al. Kinetic analysis of lesions identified on a rapid abridged multiphase (RAMP) Breast MRI protocol. Acad Radiol 2020;27(5):672–81.

35. Partridge SC, Stone KM, Strigel RM, et al. Breast DCE-MRI: influence of postcontrast timing on automated lesion kinetics assessments and discrimination of benign and malignant lesions. Acad Radiol 2014;21(9):1195–203.

36. Park KW, Han SB, Han BK, et al. MRI surveillance for women with a personal history of breast cancer: comparison between abbreviated and full diagnostic protocol. Br J Radiol 2020;93(1106): 20190733.

37. Heacock L, Gao Y, Heller SL, et al. Comparison of conventional DCE-MRI and a novel golden-angle radial multicoil compressed sensing method for the evaluation of breast lesion conspicuity. J Magn Reson Imaging 2017;45(6):1746–52.

38. Oldrini G, Fedida B, Poujol J, et al. Abbreviated breast magnetic resonance protocol: value of high-resolution temporal dynamic sequence to improve lesion characterization. Eur J Radiol 2017;95: 177–85.

39. Abe H, Mori N, Tsuchiya K, et al. Kinetic analysis of benign and malignant breast lesions with ultrafast dynamic contrast-enhanced MRI: comparison with standard kinetic assessment. AJR Am J Roentgenol 2016;207(5):1159–66.

40. Ballesio L, Savelli S, Angeletti M, et al. Breast MRI: are T2 IR sequences useful in the evaluation of breast lesions? Eur J Radiol 2009;71(1):96–101.

41. Kuhl CK, Klaschik S, Mielcarek P, et al. Do T2-weighted pulse sequences help with the differential diagnosis of enhancing lesions in dynamic breast MRI? J Magn Reson Imaging 1999;9(2):187–96.

42. Marshall H, Pham R, Sieck L, et al. Implementing abbreviated MRI screening into a breast imaging practice. AJR Am J Roentgenol 2019;1–4. https://doi.org/10.2214/AJR.18.20396.

43. Strahle DA, Pathak DR, Sierra A, et al. Systematic development of an abbreviated protocol for screening breast magnetic resonance imaging. Breast Cancer Res Treat 2017;162(2):283–95.

44. Runge VM. Critical questions regarding gadolinium deposition in the brain and body after injections of the gadolinium-based contrast agents, safety, and clinical recommendations in consideration of the EMA's pharmacovigilance and risk assessment committee recommendation for suspension of the marketing authorizations for 4 linear agents. Invest Radiol 2017;52(6):317–23.

45. Trimboli RM, Verardi N, Cartia F, et al. Breast cancer detection using double reading of unenhanced MRI including T1-weighted, T2-weighted STIR, and diffusion-weighted imaging: a proof of concept study. AJR Am J Roentgenol 2014;203(3):674–81.

46. McDonald ES, Hammersley JA, Chou SH, et al. Performance of DWI as a rapid unenhanced technique for detecting mammographically occult breast cancer in elevated-risk women with dense breasts. AJR Am J Roentgenol 2016;207(1):205–16.

47. Bickelhaupt S, Laun FB, Tesdorff J, et al. Fast and noninvasive characterization of suspicious lesions detected at breast cancer X-ray screening: capability of diffusion-weighted MR imaging with MIPs. Radiology 2016;278(3):689–97.

48. Baltzer PA, Benndorf M, Dietzel M, et al. Sensitivity and specificity of unenhanced MR mammography (DWI combined with T2-weighted TSE imaging, ueMRM) for the differentiation of mass lesions. Eur Radiol 2010;20(5):1101–10.

49. Shin HJ, Chae EY, Choi WJ, et al. Diagnostic performance of fused diffusion-weighted imaging using unenhanced or postcontrast T1-weighted MR imaging in patients with breast cancer. Medicine (Baltimore) 2016;95(17):e3502.

50. Pinker K, Moy L, Sutton EJ, et al. Diffusion-weighted imaging with apparent diffusion coefficient mapping for breast cancer detection as a stand-alone parameter: comparison with dynamic contrast-enhanced and multiparametric magnetic resonance imaging. Invest Radiol 2018;53(10):587–95.

51. Lee-Felker S, Joines M, Storer L, et al. Abbreviated Breast MRI for estimating extent of disease in newly diagnosed breast cancer. J Breast Imaging 2019; 2(1):43–9.

52. Girometti R, Nitti A, Lorenzon M, et al. Comparison between an abbreviated and full MRI protocol for detecting additional disease when doing breast cancer staging. J Magn Reson Imaging 2019; 49(7):e222–30.

53. Reig B, Heacock L, Lewin A, et al. Role of MRI to assess response to neoadjuvant therapy for breast cancer. J Magn Reson Imaging 2020. https://doi.org/10.1002/jmri.27145.

54. Kim SY, Cho N, Park IA, et al. Dynamic contrast-enhanced breast MRI for evaluating residual tumor size after neoadjuvant chemotherapy. Radiology 2018;289(2):327–34.

55. Shehata M, Grimm L, Ballantyne N, et al. Ductal carcinoma in situ: current concepts in biology, imaging, and treatment. J Breast Imaging 2019;1(3):166–76.

56. Sarwar A, Boland G, Monks A, et al. Metrics for radiologists in the era of value-based health care delivery. Radiographics 2015;35(3):866–76.

57. Borthakur A, Weinstein SP, Schnall MD, et al. Comparison of study activity times for "full" versus "fast MRI" for breast cancer screening. J Am Coll Radiol 2019;16(8):1046–51.

58. Recht MP, Block KT, Chandarana H, et al. Optimization of MRI turnaround times through the use of dockable tables and innovative architectural design strategies. AJR Am J Roentgenol 2019;212(4):855–8.

59. Dalmis MU, Gubern-Merida A, Vreemann S, et al. Artificial intelligence-based classification of breast lesions imaged with a multiparametric breast MRI protocol with ultrafast DCE-MRI, T2, and DWI. Invest Radiol 2019;54(6):325–32.

60. Johnson PM, Recht MP, Knoll F. Improving the Speed of MRI with Artificial Intelligence. Semin Musculoskelet Radiol 2020;24(1):12–20.

61. Platel B, Mus R, Welte T, et al. Automated characterization of breast lesions imaged with an ultrafast DCE-MR protocol. IEEE Trans Med Imaging 2014;33(2):225–32.

62. Petrillo A, Fusco R, Sansone M, et al. Abbreviated breast dynamic contrast-enhanced MR imaging for lesion detection and characterization: the experience of an Italian oncologic center. Breast Cancer Res Treat 2017;164(2):401–10.

63. Romeo V, Cuocolo R, Liuzzi R, et al. Preliminary results of a simplified breast MRI protocol to characterize breast lesions: comparison with a full diagnostic protocol and a review of the current literature. Acad Radiol 2017;24(11):1387–94.

64. Oldrini G, Derraz I, Salleron J, et al. Impact of an abbreviated protocol for breast MRI in diagnostic accuracy. Diagn Interv Radiol 2018;24(1):12–6.

65. Lee-Felker S, Joines M, Storer L, et al. Abbreviated breast MRI for estimating extent of disease in newly diagnosed breast cancer. Journal of Breast Imaging 2020;2(1):43–9.

Contrast-Enhanced Mammography Implementation, Performance, and Use for Supplemental Breast Cancer Screening

Matthew F. Covington, MD

KEYWORDS

- Contrast-enhanced mammography • Contrast-enhanced digital mammography
- Contrast-enhanced spectral mammography • Supplemental screening • Breast cancer
- Dense breast tissue

KEY POINTS

- Contrast-enhanced mammography (CEM) implementation and performance are discussed in detail to support new use of CEM at breast imaging centers.
- CEM may be used for a variety of indications and is recently under study to provide supplemental screening for women with dense breast tissue.
- CEM has sensitivity for cancer detection on par with contrast-enhanced breast MR imaging but has associated risks from iodinated contrast administration and radiation exposure.

INTRODUCTION

Contrast-enhanced mammography (CEM) remains an emerging technology despite being approved by the Food and Drug Administration (FDA) for clinical use since 2011. Over recent years, the number of published research studies on CEM have rapidly increased and show that CEM has sensitivity on par with MR imaging for breast cancer detection.[1,2] However, concerns regarding iodinated contrast reactions, relatively low reimbursement, current lack of commercially available direct biopsy capability, and competition with modalities like MR imaging and tomosynthesis have slowed the clinical adoption of CEM.[3,4] In 2020, CEM is considered to be a promising technology but has not yet achieved widespread usage in the breast imaging community.

Most existing publications on CEM are retrospective reviews from single imaging centers.[1,3] Larger prospective CEM trials are now on the horizon, such as the Contrast-Enhanced Mammography Imaging Screening Trial (CMIST) and the Rapid Access to Contrast-Enhanced spectral mammography in women recalled from breast cancer screening (RACER) trial.[5,6] The results of such prospective trials may determine whether CEM will ultimately achieve widespread use.

This article first presents a detailed description of CEM implementation and performance. Thereafter, use of CEM for supplemental screening is thoroughly discussed given the potential importance of this topic for the CEM community in coming years. Several thorough scientific reviews have recently been published and do not need to be repeated[1,3,7–9]; therefore, only highlights from CEM literature are discussed in this article.

Department of Radiology and Imaging Sciences, University of Utah, Center for Quantitative Cancer Imaging, Huntsman Cancer Institute, 2000 Circle of Hope, Salt Lake City, UT 84112, USA
E-mail address: matthew.covington@hsc.utah.edu

Radiol Clin N Am 59 (2021) 113–128
https://doi.org/10.1016/j.rcl.2020.08.006
0033-8389/21/© 2020 Elsevier Inc. All rights reserved.

PART 1: CONTRAST-ENHANCED MAMMOGRAPHY IMPLEMENTATION
Overview

CEM implementation is likely to be straightforward at most breast imaging centers. The physical and personnel requirements necessary for CEM implementation and performance are discussed here.

Physical Requirements for Contrast-Enhanced Mammography Imaging

CEM may be implemented in existing mammography suites as an upgrade to CEM-capable mammography systems. The ability to add CEM to existing equipment without need for additional space allocation is advantageous compared with other supplemental screening options. For CEM-capable systems, implementation requires a software upgrade from the vendor, insertion of a copper filter into the mammography unit, and access to a standard power injector.[4] If an imaging center does not have CEM-capable mammography systems, then such a system would need to be acquired. CEM-capable mammography systems are also able to perform standard mammography, tomosynthesis, and mammographic-guided or tomosynthesis-guided biopsy and localization procedures.

Although hand injection of contrast for CEM has been described in a limited number of publications,[1] a power injector for contrast administration is preferred to obtain a rapid bolus of contrast and a bolus chaser of normal saline.[1] Other physical requirements for CEM include a designated area for intravenous (IV) line insertion, designated space to monitor patients for contrast reactions, and a standard contrast reaction kit and crash cart. A portable point-of-care unit for creatinine testing is most convenient, although laboratory blood draws for creatinine testing also may be used, when indicated.

Personnel Requirements for Contrast-Enhanced Mammography Imaging

At a minimum, a radiologist and mammography technologist trained in CEM imaging are required to successfully perform CEM. Staff members must be adept with IV line placement, iodinated contrast injection, and treatment of iodinated contrast reactions. In the United States, a physician is typically required to be present when IV iodinated contrast is administered to ensure timely treatment for any severe iodinated contrast reactions.

An employee with sufficient training must screen patients for any contraindications to receive iodinated contrast. For this purpose, a radiology nurse can be particularly helpful to coordinate and assess renal function and pregnancy testing before CEM imaging, when applicable. A technologist or breast imaging nurse also may place the IV line, depending on site preference, and monitor patients for contrast reactions before the patient leaves the imaging suite.

Providing education to referring providers may promote success of a new CEM program. Referring providers should understand that CEM allows contrast-enhanced breast imaging for patients who cannot complete MR imaging for any reason, including a direct contraindication (such as a metallic implant that is not MR imaging safe), claustrophobia, patients who are too large to fit within an MR imaging scanner, or imaging expense. In addition, given rising concern regarding the safety of gadolinium contrast used in MR imaging, CEM can be presented as an option for patients and providers who prefer to avoid IV gadolinium.[10]

PART 2: CONTRAST-ENHANCED MAMMOGRAPHY PERFORMANCE

The performance of CEM requires attention to ensure patient adequacy for CEM imaging before imaging, strict adherence to image acquisition standards, and patient monitoring following CEM. An example CEM workflow is shown in **Fig. 1.**

Preparation Before Contrast-Enhanced Mammography Imaging

Before CEM imaging, a patient must be screened for any contraindication to receive IV iodinated contrast. Potential contraindications to receive IV iodinated contrast include glomerular filtration rate less than 30 mL/min per 1.73 m^2 or known allergy to iodinated contrast materials. Other exclusions to CEM imaging may include pregnancy and young patient age. It is not established whether CEM should be timed with a woman's menstrual cycle, although published literature has described performing CEM between day 5 and day 14 of the menstrual cycle.[1]

In accordance with the American College of Radiology (ACR) Manual on Contrast Media,[11] a serum creatinine measurement should be obtained in patients with 1 or more of the following: age older than 60 years, history of renal disease (including dialysis, kidney transplantation, single kidney, renal cancer, or renal surgery), hypertension requiring medical therapy, diabetes mellitus, and use of metformin or metformin-containing drugs. For these patients, a documented

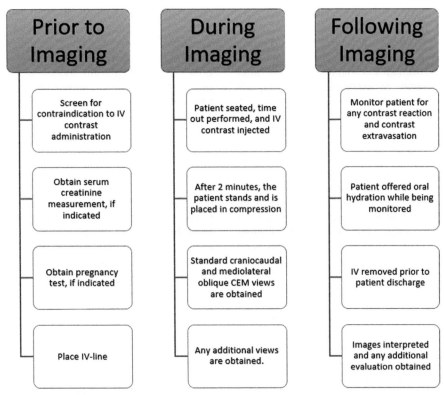

Prior to Imaging

- Screen for contraindication to IV contrast administration
- Obtain serum creatinine measurement, if indicated
- Obtain pregnancy test, if indicated
- Place IV-line

During Imaging

- Patient seated, time out performed, and IV contrast injected
- After 2 minutes, the patient stands and is placed in compression
- Standard craniocaudal and mediolateral oblique CEM views are obtained
- Any additional views are obtained.

Following Imaging

- Monitor patient for any contrast reaction and contrast extravasation
- Patient offered oral hydration while being monitored
- IV removed prior to patient discharge
- Images interpreted and any additional evaluation obtained

Fig. 1. Example CEM workflow.

creatinine value obtained within 30 days of CEM is considered sufficient if the patient's condition is stable since the last result.

Immediately before imaging, an IV must be placed. A 20-gauge needle or larger should be placed in an antecubital vein to accommodate the rapid contrast injection. A robust hand vein may also be used, if necessary. If there is a history of unilateral axillary nodal dissection, the contralateral arm is preferred for IV injection.

The patient should be informed before injection that iodinated contrast administration is frequently associated with a diffuse sensation of warmth, flushing, a metallic taste in the mouth, and urinary incontinence. In addition, the patient should be instructed to notify the technologist if there is pain during or following the injection to alert staff regarding potential contrast extravasation at the injection site.

Image Acquisition

A standard CEM examination comprises 4 low-energy views (a craniocaudal [CC] and mediolateral oblique [MLO] view of each breast) that appear nearly identical to a 2-dimensional (2D) full-field digital mammogram (FFDM). Four contrast-enhanced recombined views in the same projections are also obtained simultaneously. Additional diagnostic views, including spot compression views, also may be obtained as tailored for individual case.[4] All CEM images are taken after the IV administration of iodinated contrast material (such as Iohexol or equivalent, 1.5 mL/kg) that is typically injected at a rate of 3 mL/s followed by an additional 10-mL saline flush.

An example workflow may have an IV placed by a nurse or technologist, after which time the patient is seated in the mammography suite, a time out is performed, the IV line is connected to the power injector, a tight seal between the power injector line and IV tubing is confirmed, and the IV is assessed for patency with a saline flush. Contrast is thereafter injected through the IV, and the patient remains seated as contrast washes into the breast for 2 minutes. During this time, the patient should be monitored for any signs of contrast extravasation or any early contrast reaction. After 2 minutes, the technologist positions the patient and obtains all views within a window of 2 to 6 minutes following contrast injection for a total imaging time of approximately 8 to 10 minutes.[4]

CEM imaging should begin no earlier than 2 minutes after IV contrast administration to allow adequate time for contrast to wash into the breast. The patient's breast should not be in compression during the initial 2 minutes after contrast injection, as compression will impede blood flow and limit contrast entry into the breast. There is no universal standard as to whether imaging should begin 2 minutes after the start of contrast administration or 2 minutes after the completion of contrast administration. It is possible that imaging at 2 minutes after the completion of contrast administration allows slightly more time for contrast to enter the breast, which could improve the conspicuity of contrast enhancement within breast lesions. Further research is necessary to determine if there is an advantage to either of these approaches.

Several strategies exist to make certain all desired images are obtained within 6 minutes after contrast injection. First, each case should be reviewed in advance to determine whether any views in addition to the standard CC and MLO views of each breast should be obtained. For example, if a lesion is in the far lateral and posterior breast, an exaggerated CC view could be requested in advance. Second, having a more experienced technologist position and obtain images may allow extra time for additional images to be obtained and reduce the likelihood that an image may need to be repeated for technical reasons. Depending on availability, having 2 technologists in the room can be beneficial to allow the first technologist to focus solely on positioning while the other technologist readies and performs contrast injection and image acquisition on the mammography control console. Last, having the radiologist directly in the mammography imaging suite at time of imaging can allow the radiologist to review images as they are obtained and direct the technologist as to whether any views need to be repeated or if any additional views need to be obtained based on review of imaging in real-time. Alternatively, the radiologist could review images in the reading room immediately after they are obtained and direct the technologist(s) regarding any need to obtain additional views.

Contrast-Enhanced Mammography Views

Contrast-enhanced recombined images are obtained through a dual-energy logarithmic subtraction technique that removes breast parenchymal tissue from the image and provides an image that highlights areas of contrast enhancement. The dual-energy technique obtains the low-energy image (26–32 kVp) and then a high-energy image

(44–50 kVp) that straddles the 33.2 keV k-edge of iodine.[1,3] These images are obtained in rapid succession while the breast is held in the same compression. Low-energy images and recombined postcontrast images are subsequently sent to a picture archiving and communication system for interpretation. The high-energy images are not included for image interpretation but are rather obtained solely to allow for logarithmic subtraction, and neither the low nor high energy depict areas of contrast enhancement. Compared with 2D FFDM and tomosynthesis, CEM derives diagnostic advantage from the removal of breast parenchymal tissue via logarithmic subtraction and the administration of iodinated contrast materials that highlight areas of increased blood flow via tumor-induced angiogenesis. Like contrast-enhanced breast MR imaging, this technique overcomes the masking effect of dense breast tissue on a standard mammogram that facilitates detection of mammographic-occult and tomosynthesis-occult cancers.

A CC and MLO view of each breast should be routinely obtained for a CEM examination, analogous to routinely imaging each breast for a breast MR imaging study. Both CEM and MR imaging demonstrate variable degrees of background parenchymal enhancement and comparison of the intensity and extent of enhancement in each breast is necessary to assess for background enhancement versus pathologic enhancement in each breast.

No current standard exists as to the order of which CEM views should be obtained.[1] However, obtaining images in a consistent pattern may aid the interpretation of a CEM study. For example, if one routinely obtains MLO views of each breast first, followed by CC views, then MLO views will routinely represent an earlier phase of enhancement than CC views, allowing a rough albeit not-as-yet validated assessment of enhancement kinetics within a mass. In such a scenario, if a mass demonstrated robust enhancement on the MLO images obtained first, compared with the CC images obtained later, one could suppose that rapid arterial enhancement with washout may be present. Others have looked at the degree of enhancement on CEM as a predictor of malignancy, with strong enhancement being more predictive of malignant lesions.[12,13]

Note that formal kinetic assessment is theoretically possible with CEM but is not performed due to the multiple radiation exposures that would result from obtaining sequential images in the same projection over time. Obtaining views of each breast in the same projection before proceeding with another projection (for example an

MLO view of each breast before obtaining CC views) will maximally ensure that a corresponding pair of images is available for each breast if imaging is terminated early for any reason. An example workflow for image acquisition is shown in **Fig. 2**. If the degree of contrast enhancement in the breast appears weaker than expected on initial images (such as when performing extent of disease evaluation for a known[14] malignancy) the first view(s) could be repeated at the end of the study to assess for improved depiction of enhancement on more delayed imaging.

A combination mode wherein tomosynthesis and CEM images are obtained simultaneously in the same breast compression may be performed. In such a scenario, approximately 2 minutes after IV contrast injection, a tomosynthesis image set may first be obtained, followed by the low-energy and high-energy images of CEM, thereby providing tomosynthesis, low-energy, and subtracted images coregistered from the same compression for direct comparison and review. Imaging that provides 3D assessment of contrast enhancement, or that overlies contrast-enhanced images on tomosynthesis slices, is not currently available. One must be cognizant of the added radiation to the patient from performing tomosynthesis in addition to CEM, as this will result in 3 separate exposures to ionizing radiation per view obtained. In a 2017 phantom study, the average glandular dose per view at a mean phantom breast thickness of 63 mm was 3.0 mGy for CEM compared with 2.1 mGy for 2D FFDM and 2.5 mGy for tomosynthesis.[14] Therefore, the addition of simultaneous tomosynthesis to a CEM study may increase the average glandular dose by approximately 80% (5.5 mGy compared with 3.0 mGy).

After Contrast-Enhanced Mammography Imaging

After imaging, a patient should be monitored for any contrast reaction or extravasation. Duration of monitoring may vary depending on site preference but should be at least 15 minutes after imaging. The patient should be given instructions regarding subsequent self-monitoring for any contrast reaction and be given appropriate follow-up instructions should this manifest. In addition, the patient may be given fluids to hydrate after imaging. The IV line should remain in place until shortly before the patient is discharged because IV access may be needed if a severe contrast reaction develops.

PART 3: CONTRAST-ENHANCED MAMMOGRAPHY INTERPRETATION

CEM images may be interpreted by the radiologist while the patient is still present, facilitating additional imaging evaluation when necessary, or images may be interpreted after the patient has left the imaging suite. At present, most CEM examinations are performed for diagnostic evaluation rather than screening, and immediate reads may be preferred in that setting.[4,15] However, if CEM were used for high-risk screening, standard CC and MLO views of each breast could be obtained by the technologist(s) and either immediate or delayed reads could be performed.

CEM interpretation may have a low learning curve for breast imagers because CEM blends the interpretation standards and reporting lexicon of mammography and contrast-enhanced breast MR imaging.[16,17] A CEM report should contain a description of breast density based on the low-energy (2D FFDM-like) images according to the current recommendations of the ACR Breast

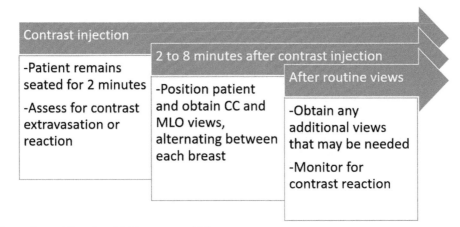

Fig. 2. Example workflow for CEM image acquisition.

Imaging-Reporting and Data System (BI-RADS) Atlas.[18,19] Like breast MR imaging, the degree of background parenchymal enhancement based off the recombined postcontrast images should be reported as minimal, mild, moderate, or marked.[20] An example CEM reporting template is shown in **Fig. 3**.

Low-energy CEM images have been shown to be noninferior to 2D FFDM views for mammographic interpretation.[21] A CEM report should describe typical mammographic findings based on the low-energy images in terms of masses, microcalcifications, architectural distortion, asymmetries, and so forth, according to standard BI-RADS recommendations for mammographic imaging.[19] If concurrent tomosynthesis imaging was performed, any tomosynthesis findings should be reported along with low-energy CEM imaging findings.

Recombined postcontrast images may be reported following the MR imaging reporting lexicon from BI-RADS.[16,17,20,22] Evaluation of the recombined postcontrast images includes assessment of abnormal areas of enhancement in terms of foci, masses, and nonmass enhancement as in breast MR imaging.[20] When appropriate, size measurements may be reported separately for the low-energy and recombined postcontrast images, or in unison if there is agreement. Prior studies have shown that the size measurements of a lesion on CEM are comparable to those of MR imaging.[23,24]

Finally, a BI-RADS assessment category and appropriate follow-up recommendations should be reported, according to the standard BI-RADS lexicon.[25] A site also may choose to include details regarding type and amount of IV contrast and the patient's creatinine and glomerular filtration rate values in the clinical report.

PART 4: FURTHER MANAGEMENT OF CONTRAST-ENHANCED MAMMOGRAPHY IMAGING FINDINGS
Further Evaluation of Suspicious Contrast-Enhanced Mammography Lesions

Any new suspicious finding identified on CEM images should be assessed with recent or follow-up

---

HISTORY:

COMPARISON:

TECHNIQUE: Full field digital mammographic views were performed including low energy and recombined views following the intravenous administration of iodinated contrast material.

Estimated GFR:
Creatinine:
Contrast:

BREAST PARENCHYMAL COMPOSITION:

FINDINGS:

Low energy images:

No suspicious masses, calcifications, or areas of architectural distortion are seen.

OR

There is a (finding description) in the (LEFT or RIGHT) breast (location) (measuring).

Post-contrast recombined images:

Background enhancement: (minimal, mild, moderate or marked) (symmetric or asymmetric)

No suspicious mass or non-mass enhancement is seen.

OR

There is a (mild, moderate OR markedly) enhancing (mass OR region of non-mass enhancement) in the (LEFT or RIGHT) breast (location) (measuring).

IMPRESSION:

OVERALL FINAL ASSESSMENT: BIRADS (0 to 6)

RECOMMENDATION:

Fig. 3. Example template for CEM reporting.

diagnostic mammography and ultrasound to establish benignity, or else identify a target for follow-up or biopsy.[26] For most cases, a corresponding target will be evident on additional diagnostic views and/or CEM-directed ultrasound. A potential advantage of CEM compared with MR imaging is that the location of CEM enhancement on standard CC and MLO views is easier to correlate on additional mammogram and ultrasound view compared with MR imaging that is not obtained in mammographic imaging planes. When a correlating lesion is biopsied, the clip location on postbiopsy mammography may be directly compared with the location of CEM enhancement to assess for appropriate tissue sampling. Determining exact positional concordance between postbiopsy mammogram and MR imaging is less accurate.

Depicting the location and extent of abnormal contrast enhancement on CEM also allows direct comparison with mammography at time of mammographic localization for presurgical bracketing. Extrapolating the extent of abnormal enhancement seen on MR imaging to a mammogram for presurgical localization or bracketing is not as easy given that MR imaging has different positioning compared with mammography.

Suspicious CEM enhancement should be correlated with diagnostic mammography, tomosynthesis, and/or targeted ultrasound to identify a biopsy target. If no biopsy target is seen on these modalities, contrast-enhanced breast MR imaging would then be necessary for further evaluation and to guide subsequent biopsy, if indicated.

Biopsy of Suspicious Contrast-Enhanced Mammography Lesions

Current CEM systems are not capable of biopsy with direct CEM guidance, although a CEM biopsy system has been announced by at least 1 vendor, pending FDA 510k approval.[27] Several workaround options exist whereby the CEM-detected lesions may ultimately be sampled. The first option is to biopsy a correlating lesion using ultrasound, tomosynthesis, or stereotactic biopsy. In certain cases, finding a tomosynthesis correlate may be aided by obtaining coregistered tomosynthesis images at time of CEM imaging. If no correlating lesion is identified on mammogram or ultrasound, MR imaging should be performed to identify a corresponding lesion for MR imaging–guided biopsy. If no lesion is seen on MR imaging, then short-interval CEM follow-up rather than biopsy may be indicated.

A method has been described whereby a lesion may first be localized under direct CEM guidance

for placement of a biopsy clip, radioactive seed, or other localization device at the area of abnormal CEM enhancement; subsequently, biopsy targeting the clip or seed may be performed using tomosynthesis or stereotactic biopsy versus surgical excisional biopsy.[4]

PART 5: POTENTIAL USE OF CONTRAST-ENHANCED MAMMOGRAPHY FOR SUPPLEMENTAL SCREENING

Multiple comprehensive CEM literature reviews have recently been published.[1,3,7–9,26] To date, CEM has been evaluated for many uses including presurgical evaluation for extent of disease and staging of known malignancy[2,23,28–38] (Fig. 4), neoadjuvant therapy response monitoring,[24,39–41] abnormal findings on screening mammography/complicated mammography troubleshooting,[42–48] imaging of patients with an MR imaging contraindication,[31] symptomatic breast evaluation,[15,44,49,50] evaluation of indeterminate mammographic calcifications,[48,51,52] evaluation of mammographic architectural distortion[53] (Fig. 5), mammographic imaging for women with dense breast tissue and/or high-risk supplemental screening[30,54,55] (Fig. 6), to reduce biopsy rate for low to moderate suspicion soft tissue lesions,[56] and postoperative breast cancer surveillance.[57]

Supplemental screening is of great interest to the breast cancer community because the sensitivity of routine screening mammography is reduced in women with dense breast tissue due to a masking effect of dense tissue that can obscure a cancer on a mammogram.[26,58] Dense breast tissue is common, and 40% to 50% of women in the screening population are estimated to have dense breast tissue.[58,59] Considering that at least 40 million screening mammograms are performed each year in the United States, 16 to 20 million supplemental screening examinations would be performed annually if supplemental screening were universally implemented.[58,60] To best provide supplemental screening for this large number of women, a supplemental screening examination must be inexpensive, safe, highly accessible, and demonstrate a high sensitivity for cancer detection.

CEM is inexpensive compared with MR imaging,[61] and CEM is typically reimbursed as the cost of a diagnostic mammogram plus a small additional charge (approximately $35) for contrast administration. However, unlike MR imaging or ultrasound,[62] CEM uses ionizing radiation and requires the intravenous injection of iodinated contrast. Although it is unclear whether added cost or an IV contrast-enhanced examination will

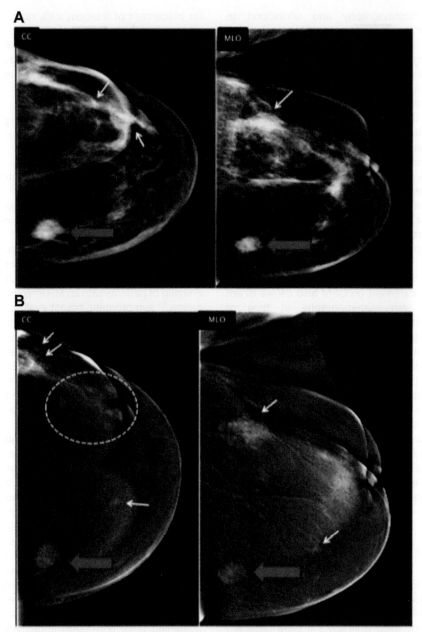

Fig. 4. A 53-year-old woman with prior left breast conservation surgery 1 year before presenting with a new palpable lower inner quadrant area of concern. (*A*) Traditional digital mammograms in the craniocaudal and mediolateral oblique views showed a malignant-looking mass with spiculated margins (*thick arrow*) in the lower inner quadrant. In addition, there are suspicious asymmetries within the operative bed (*small arrows*). (*B*) CEM recombined postcontrast images confirm abnormal enhancement in the lower inner quadrant mass and reveal multiple enhancing foci and upper outer quadrant nonmass enhancement about the postsurgical scar. In this case, CEM not only confirmed the diagnosis of malignancy but also displayed a more extensive distribution of disease, shown to represent multicentric invasive ductal carcinoma. (*From* Helal MH, Mansour SM, Ahmed HA, et al. The role of contrast-enhanced spectral mammography in the evaluation of the postoperative breast cancer. *Clin Radiol.* 2019;74(10):771-781; with permission.)

A   **B**   **C**

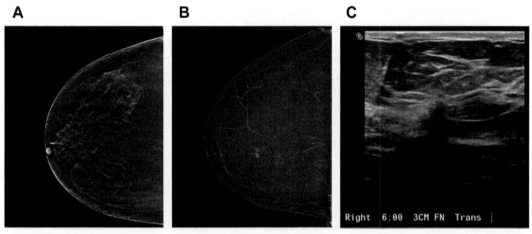

Fig. 5. A 59-year-old woman with architectural distortion. (*A*) FFCT shows architectural distortion in the central breast, deep to the nipple. (*B*) Recombined postcontrast CC image shows enhancement within the lesion. (*C*) Ultrasound of the lesion shows a small, shadowing mass. The lesion was a biopsy-proven invasive ductal carcinoma. (*From* Patel BK, Naylor ME, Kosiorek HE, et al. Clinical utility of contrast-enhanced spectral mammography as an adjunct for tomosynthesis-directed architectural distortion. *Clin Imaging*. 2017;46:44-52; with permission.)

be acceptable to most patients presenting for supplemental screening, a recent survey of women with dense breast tissue suggested that obtaining an imaging study with high sensitivity would outweigh added cost as well as a need for IV line placement.[63]

To date, the most common options for supplemental screening are whole breast ultrasound and tomosynthesis, both of which demonstrate lower sensitivity for cancer detection compared with MR imaging.[59,64] Other emerging options for supplemental screening include molecular breast imaging[65] and CEM.[66–68] See **Table 1** for comparison of current emerging supplemental screening options.

Diagnostic Performance of Contrast-Enhanced Mammography for Supplemental Screening

Based on 2 studies, CEM demonstrates an overall cancer detection rate of 15.5 in women at intermediate and high lifetime risk of development of breast malignancy[66] and an incremental cancer detection rate of 13.1 in women at intermediate risk of development of breast malignancy[68] cancers per 1000 women undergoing supplemental screening. CEM also demonstrates sensitivity reported at 87.5%[66] and 90.5%,[68] specificity reported at 93.7%[66] and 76.1%,[68] and negative predictive values of 99.7%[66] and 99.6%[68] when used for supplemental screening.

For comparison, incremental cancer detection rates over traditional mammography have been estimated to be 4.4 per 1000 examinations for ultrasound and up to 2.5 per 1000 examinations

for tomosynthesis.[69] Recent studies on breast MR imaging for supplemental screening have reported incremental cancer detection rates of 16.5 cancers[70] and 11.8 cancers[71] per 1000 examinations.

CEM, as with all supplemental screening options, will demonstrate false positive findings that may lead to additional imaging and biopsy for benign findings. Larger prospective trials are necessary to further understand the diagnostic performance, feasibility, and best use of CEM for supplemental screening. The prospective CMIST trial is already planned.[5] Prospective trials that directly compare CEM along with other supplemental screening options to include ultrasound, molecular breast imaging, and/or MR imaging would also be helpful.

Safety of Iodinated Contrast Administration

Risks of severe hypersensitivity reactions to iodinated contrast may occur in up to 4 in 10,000 IV administrations (0.04%) with 0 to 10 deaths per every million administrations based on data from other imaging studies.[11,72,73] A recent CEM literature review estimated an overall adverse event rate of a contrast reaction during CEM imaging of 0.82% (95% confidence interval 0.64%–1.05%) with only a single reaction of 30 being severe but nonfatal.[1]

If supplemental screening with CEM was performed for 16 to 20 million US women annually, and the overall risk of iodinated contrast reactions of any severity is 0.82%, this corresponds with 131,200 to 164,000 contrast reactions

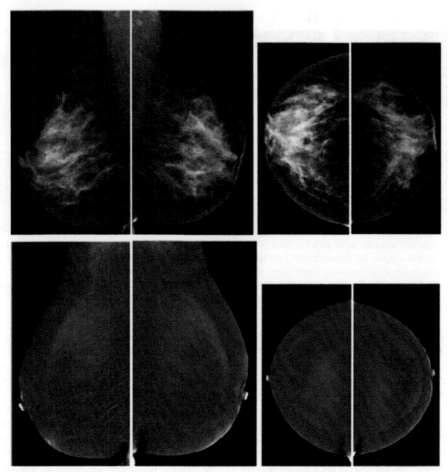

Fig. 6. A 45-year-old woman at high risk for breast cancer development presented for annual screening mammography. Low-energy (*top row*) and recombined postcontrast (*bottom row*) mediolateral oblique and craniocaudal images of both breasts are provided. Low-energy images show heterogeneously dense breast parenchyma, which may obscure small masses. No abnormal areas of enhancement are seen in either breast on recombined postcontrast images, confirming that no mass is obscured by the dense breast tissue. (*From* Bhimani C, Matta D, Roth RG, et al. Contrast-enhanced spectral mammography: technique, indications, and clinical applications. *Acad Radiol.* 2017;24:84-88; with permission.)

annually, most of which would be mild reactions. If the rate of severe contrast reactions is 0.04%, this would result in 6400 to 8000 severe contrast reactions per year from the 16 to 20 million CEM studies performed. Finally, if 0 to 10 deaths per 1 million iodinated contrast administrations is predicted, 0 to 200 women per year in the United States could experience a fatal contrast reaction from 16 to 20 million CEM supplemental screening studies.

The estimated risk of severe iodinated contrast reaction is therefore very small for any individual patient undergoing CEM supplemental screening but becomes more significant on the population level. For women undergoing supplemental screening, however, the mortality risk of undetected breast cancer is certain to outweigh the

mortality risk of iodinated contrast reactions, but further evaluation is necessary to refine and establish risk estimates. When evaluating the safety profile of CEM compared with less-sensitive supplemental screening options such as ultrasound or tomosynthesis, one must remember that the failure of supplemental screening to identify a cancer poses theoretic mortality risk.

IV injection of iodinated contrast also has been assumed to cause contrast-induced nephropathy in select patients, although the occurrence and risk of contrast-induced nephropathy is now controversial.[74] Nevertheless, CEM should be performed in concordance with current ACR practice parameters in terms of ensuring adequate renal function before IV contrast administration.[11] Alternative imaging modalities may be pursued for

Table 1
Comparison of current and emerging supplemental screening modalities

Imaging Modality	Relative Incremental Cancer Detection Rate	Need for IV Placement	Potential for Contrast Reactions	Relative Average Radiation Exposure	Interpretation Time	Imaging Time	Cost
Contrast-enhanced mammography	***	Yes	***	*	*	**	**
Automated whole breast ultrasound	**	No	None	None	***	***	*
Hand-held whole breast ultrasound	**	No	None	None	*	***	*
Molecular breast imaging	***	Yes	None	**	*	***	**
Abbreviated breast MR imaging	****	Yes	*	None	**	**	Undetermined
Standard breast MR imaging	****	Yes	*	None	****	****	****

For pertinent columns, examinations are compared on a scale of 1 to 4 asterisks, with single asterisks denoting the lowest relative value and 4 asterisks denoting the highest relative value.
Abbreviation: IV, intravenous.

those patients whose renal function does not permit IV contrast administration for CEM.

Safety of Ionizing Radiation Exposure

CEM exposes patients to ionizing radiation with theoretic risks of cancer induction, even at low doses. Available literature on CEM radiation doses is scarce, but average glandular doses are reported in a recent literature review to range from 1.5 to 6.9 mGy per examination and 0.43 to 2.7 mGy per view.[1] Most of the radiation dose is received from the low-energy exposure given higher absorbed doses of radiation with lower kVp exposures. Performing simultaneous tomosynthesis with CEM will further increase the dose of each examination. As previously mentioned, a 2017 phantom study reported that the average glandular dose per view at a mean phantom breast thickness of 63 mm was 3.0 mGy for CEM compared with 2.1 mGy for 2D FFDM and 2.5 mGy for tomosynthesis.[14]

Formal benefit-to-radiation risk calculations have not been performed for CEM supplemental screening use due to the paucity of literature. However, results of prospective trials such as CMIST may provide information necessary to obtain such benefit-to-risk estimates and further inform the appropriate use of CEM for supplemental screening.

One potential strategy that would reduce the additional radiation exposure from CEM for supplemental screening is to allow CEM to substitute for routine screening mammography for women with dense breast tissue.[4] Under this strategy, routine screening with 2D FFDM and/or tomosynthesis would not be performed and CEM would be the only annual screening examination performed. This should theoretically be possible because the low-energy images from CEM may substitute for standard mammographic screening,[21] and the recombined postcontrast images would provide supplemental screening by removing dense breast tissue from the image and providing assessment of any abnormal enhancement. Beyond lowering total radiation exposure, this single-examination screening strategy also would be more convenient for women, which would foster adherence to supplemental screening and reduce costs compared with other supplemental screening options that require 2 separate examinations (routine screening mammogram and a subsequent supplemental screening examination) to be performed.

Cost Considerations of Contrast-Enhanced Mammography for Supplemental Screening

CEM acquisition costs are typically low, as CEM is typically available as a software upgrade to most current mammography systems. CEM is typically reimbursed at the same rate as a diagnostic mammogram with a small additional charge for contrast materials. For this and other reasons, CEM total imaging costs are estimated to be approximately 25% that of MR imaging.[61] This low cost of imaging may be simultaneously advantageous and an impediment for CEM adoption depending on the scenario for which CEM is considered.

On one hand, CEM may provide lower-cost contrast-enhanced imaging for patients for whom MR imaging is not considered cost-effective, such as women with dense breast tissue who are otherwise not at high risk. Screening breast MR imaging is currently considered cost-effective only for women at greater than 20% lifetime risk of breast malignancy, or with a known condition for which the prevalence of breast cancer is greater than 1% to 3%.[75,76] Therefore, women with dense breast tissue typically cannot obtain insurance coverage for supplemental screening MR imaging. At present, CEM typically does not have the same preauthorization requirements and restrictive insurance coverage found with breast MR imaging. Women with dense breast tissue but no other risk factors are therefore more likely to have CEM covered by insurers. Abbreviated MR imaging protocols that may lower the cost of MR imaging are under study and have shown promise for supplemental screening, although it remains unclear whether insurers will cover this examination for dense breast tissue supplemental screening.[71,77,78]

On the other hand, the relatively low reimbursement of CEM is an impediment to CEM adoption if CEM will be performed in lieu of more lucrative MR imaging. For example, if CEM were to replace MR imaging for extent of disease evaluation, imaging practices would generate much less revenue due to the differential reimbursement of these studies. However, If CEM is performed for indications that do not compete with MR imaging, such as supplemental screening for women at average to intermediate risk of breast cancer, CEM would generate positive revenue. If future payment models shift away from fee-for-service to cost-sharing models,[79] CEM would become increasingly attractive for imaging centers and hospital systems.

CEM-capable mammography systems can also be used for high-volume mammographic screening, diagnostic mammography, and stereotactic and/or tomosynthesis biopsy, and these multiple revenue streams may help justify the cost of purchase compared with other single-use supplemental screening technologies, such as automated whole breast ultrasound.

PART 6: FUTURE DIRECTIONS

An opportunity exists to study use of artificial intelligence and machine learning with CEM. A feasibility study using computer-aided diagnosis from machine-learning algorithms showed that the computer-aided diagnostic tool provided useful information to radiologists that allowed a reduction in false positive findings.[80] An opportunity also exists to use machine learning to predict which women with dense breast tissue are most likely to benefit from supplemental screening to thereafter target supplemental screening to those women most likely to benefit. Finally, direct comparisons of CEM with other supplemental screening options such as whole breast ultrasound and molecular breast imaging are also needed.

SUMMARY

This article provides an overview of the implementation and performance of CEM, and potential use of CEM for supplemental screening. In summary, CEM is a highly sensitive and relatively low-cost breast imaging examination that has yet to find widespread use among breast imagers. Most of the potential indications for CEM overlap with contrast-enhanced breast MR imaging and a unique indication that cannot be addressed by MR imaging has yet to be established. However, CEM is of obvious utility when MR imaging cannot be performed due to an MR imaging contraindication, claustrophobia, desire to avoid gadolinium exposure, or cost. Given that breast MR imaging is currently not considered cost-effective for supplemental screening of women with dense breast tissue at average lifetime risk, CEM may be able to address this need. CEM could be studied as a stand-alone screening option for women with dense breast tissue, obviating the need for standard screening mammography in addition to a supplemental screening examination.

CLINICS CARE POINTS

- Early studies evaluating CEM use for supplemental screening are promising and additional prospective trials are on the horizon.
- CEM implementation should be straightforward for most breast imaging centers given favorable physical and personnel requirements.
- CEM image interpretation blends the reporting standards of mammography and breast MR imaging and is likely to have a low learning curve for experienced breast imagers.
- CEM is under study for supplemental breast cancer screening as postcontrast recombined images remove dense breast from the image and show presence of lack of abnormal enhancement, thereby overcoming the masking effect of dense breast tissue on standard mammography.
- If used for supplemental screening, CEM must balance the benefit of incremental cancer detection with risks of iodinated contrast reaction and exposure to ionizing radiation.
- CEM adoption is not yet widespread, but results of upcoming prospective trials may accelerate adoption of this technology.

DISCLOSURE

Dr M.F. Covington is a consultant for Hologic, Inc. for educational speaking on contrast-enhanced mammography.

REFERENCES

1. Zanardo M, Cozzi A, Trimboli RM, et al. Technique, protocols and adverse reactions for contrast-enhanced spectral mammography (CESM): a systematic review. Insights Imaging 2019;10(1):76.
2. Sumkin JH, Berg WA, Carter GJ, et al. Diagnostic performance of MRI, molecular breast imaging, and contrast-enhanced mammography in women with newly diagnosed breast cancer. Radiology 2019;293(3):531–40.
3. Lewin JM, Patel BK, Tanna A. Contrast-enhanced mammography: a scientific review. J Breast Imaging 2019;2(1):7–15.
4. Covington MF, Pizzitola VJ, Lorans R, et al. The future of contrast-enhanced mammography. AJR Am J Roentgenol 2018;210(2):292–300.
5. American College of Radiology. Contrast enhanced mammography imaging screening trial (CMIST) 2020. Available at: https://www.acr.org/Research/Clinical-Research/CMIST. Accessed April 28, 2020.
6. Neeter L, Houben IPL, Nelemans PJ, et al. Rapid Access to Contrast-Enhanced spectral mammoGRaphy in women recalled from breast cancer screening: the RACER trial study design. Trials 2019;20(1):759.
7. Patel BK, Lobbes MBI, Lewin J. Contrast enhanced spectral mammography: a review. Semin Ultrasound CT MR 2018;39(1):70–9.
8. Tagliafico AS, Bignotti B, Rossi F, et al. Diagnostic performance of contrast-enhanced spectral mammography: systematic review and meta-analysis. Breast 2016;28:13–9.
9. Zhu X, Huang JM, Zhang K, et al. Diagnostic value of contrast-enhanced spectral mammography for screening breast cancer: systematic review and

meta-analysis. Clin Breast Cancer 2018;18(5): e985–95.

10. Cozzi A, Schiaffino S, Sardanelli F. The emerging role of contrast-enhanced mammography. Quant Imaging Med Surg 2019;9(12):2012–8.

11. American College of Radiology Committee on Drugs and Contrast Media. ACR manual on contrast media 2020. Available at: https://www.acr.org/-/media/ACR/Files/Clinical-Resources/Contrast_Media.pdf. Accessed April 28, 2020.

12. Rudnicki W, Heinze S, Piegza T, et al. Correlation between enhancement intensity in contrast enhancement spectral mammography and types of kinetic curves in magnetic resonance imaging. Med Sci Monit 2020;26:e920742.

13. Rudnicki W, Heinze S, Niemiec J, et al. Correlation between quantitative assessment of contrast enhancement in contrast-enhanced spectral mammography (CESM) and histopathology-preliminary results. Eur Radiol 2019;29(11): 6220–6.

14. James JR, Pavlicek W, Hanson JA, et al. Breast radiation dose with CESM compared with 2D FFDM and 3D tomosynthesis mammography. AJR Am J roentgenology 2017;208(2):362–72.

15. Lewis TC, Pizzitola VJ, Giurescu ME, et al. Contrast-enhanced digital mammography: a single-institution experience of the first 208 cases. Breast J 2017; 23(1):67–76.

16. Knogler T, Homolka P, Hoernig M, et al. Application of BI-RADS descriptors in contrast-enhanced dual-energy mammography: comparison with MRI. Breast Care (Basel) 2017;12(4):212–6.

17. Travieso-Aja MM, Maldonado-Saluzzi D, Naranjo-Santana P, et al. Evaluation of the applicability of BI-RADS(R) MRI for the interpretation of contrast-enhanced digital mammography. Radiologia 2019; 61(6):477–88.

18. Radiology ACo. ACR BI-RADS Atlas part II. Reporting System. 2013. Available at: https://www.acr.org/-/media/ACR/Files/RADS/BI-RADS/Mammography-Reporting.pdf. Accessed April 29, 2020.

19. Sickles EA, D'Orsi CJ, Bassett LW, et al. ACR BI-RADS® mammography. In: D'Orsi CJ, editor. ACR BI-RADS® atlas, breast imaging reporting and data system. Reston (VA): American College of Radiology; 2013. p. 171–5.

20. Morris EA, Comstock CE, Lee CH, et al. ACR BI-RADS® magnetic resonance imaging. In: D'Orsi CJ, editor. ACR BI-RADS® atlas, breast imaging reporting and data system. Reston (VA): American College of Radiology; 2013. p. 23–4.

21. Lalji UC, Jeukens CR, Houben I, et al. Evaluation of low-energy contrast-enhanced spectral mammography images by comparing them to full-field digital mammography using EUREF image quality criteria. Eur Radiol 2015;25(10):2813–20.

22. Kamal RM, Helal MH, Mansour SM, et al. Can we apply the MRI BI-RADS lexicon morphology descriptors on contrast-enhanced spectral mammography? Br J Radiol 2016;89(1064):20160157.

23. Lobbes MB, Lalji UC, Nelemans PJ, et al. The quality of tumor size assessment by contrast-enhanced spectral mammography and the benefit of additional breast MRI. J Cancer 2015;6(2):144–50.

24. Patel BK, Hilal T, Covington M, et al. Contrast-enhanced spectral mammography is comparable to MRI in the assessment of residual breast cancer following neoadjuvant systemic therapy. Ann Surg Oncol 2018;25(5):1350–6.

25. D'Orsi CJ SE, Mendelson EB, Morris EA, et al. ACR BI-RADS® atlas, breast imaging reporting and data system. Reston (VA): American College of Radiology; 2013.

26. Ghaderi KF, Phillips J, Perry H, et al. Contrast-enhanced mammography: current applications and future directions. Radiographics 2019;39(7):1907–20.

27. U.S. Food & Drug Administration. 510(k) premarket notification 2020. Available at: https://www.accessdata.fda.gov/scripts/cdrh/cfdocs/cfPMN/pmn.cfm?start_search=1&productcode=MUE&knumber=&applicant=GE%20HEALTHCARE. Accessed May 27, 2020.

28. Ali-Mucheru M, Pockaj B, Patel B, et al. Contrast-enhanced digital mammography in the surgical management of breast cancer. Ann Surg Oncol 2016;23(Suppl 5):649–55.

29. Lee-Felker SA, Tekchandani L, Thomas M, et al. Newly diagnosed breast cancer: comparison of contrast-enhanced spectral mammography and breast MR imaging in the evaluation of extent of disease. Radiology 2017;285(2):389–400.

30. Patel BK, Garza SA, Eversman S, et al. Assessing tumor extent on contrast-enhanced spectral mammography versus full-field digital mammography and ultrasound. Clin Imaging 2017;46: 78–84.

31. Richter V, Hatterman V, Preibsch H, et al. Contrast-enhanced spectral mammography in patients with MRI contraindications. Acta Radiol 2018;59(7): 798–805.

32. Fallenberg EM, Dromain C, Diekmann F, et al. Contrast-enhanced spectral mammography: does mammography provide additional clinical benefits or can some radiation exposure be avoided? Breast Cancer Res Treat 2014;146(2):371–81.

33. Patel BK, Davis J, Ferraro C, et al. Value added of preoperative contrast-enhanced digital mammography in patients with invasive lobular carcinoma of the breast. Clin Breast Cancer 2018;18(6): e1339–45.

34. Travieso-Aja MDM, Naranjo-Santana P, Fernandez-Ruiz C, et al. Factors affecting the precision of lesion

sizing with contrast-enhanced spectral mammography. Clin Radiol 2018;73(3):296–303.

35. Helal MH, Mansour SM, Salaleldin LA, et al. The impact of contrast-enhanced spectral mammogram (CESM) and three-dimensional breast ultrasound (3DUS) on the characterization of the disease extend in cancer patients. Br J Radiol 2018; 91(1087):20170977.

36. Helal MH, Mansour SM, Zaglol M, et al. Staging of breast cancer and the advanced applications of digital mammogram: what the physician needs to know? Br J Radiol 2017;90(1071):20160717.

37. Ambicka A, Luczynska E, Adamczyk A, et al. The tumour border on contrast-enhanced spectral mammography and its relation to histological characteristics of invasive breast cancer. Pol J Pathol 2016;67(3):295–9.

38. Blum KS, Rubbert C, Mathys B, et al. Use of contrast-enhanced spectral mammography for intra-mammary cancer staging: preliminary results. Acad Radiol 2014;21(11):1363–9.

39. Iotti V, Ravaioli S, Vacondio R, et al. Contrast-enhanced spectral mammography in neoadjuvant chemotherapy monitoring: a comparison with breast magnetic resonance imaging. Breast Cancer Res 2017;19(1):106.

40. Barra FR, de Souza FF, Camelo R, et al. Accuracy of contrast-enhanced spectral mammography for estimating residual tumor size after neoadjuvant chemotherapy in patients with breast cancer: a feasibility study. Radiol Bras 2017;50(4):224–30.

41. Barra FR, Sobrinho AB, Barra RR, et al. Contrast-enhanced mammography (CEM) for detecting residual disease after neoadjuvant chemotherapy: a comparison with breast magnetic resonance imaging (MRI). Biomed Res Int 2018;2018:8531916.

42. Houben IPL, Van de Voorde P, Jeukens C, et al. Contrast-enhanced spectral mammography as work-up tool in patients recalled from breast cancer screening has low risks and might hold clinical benefits. Eur J Radiol 2017;94:31–7.

43. Lobbes MB, Lalji U, Houwers J, et al. Contrast-enhanced spectral mammography in patients referred from the breast cancer screening programme. Eur Radiol 2014;24(7):1668–76.

44. Chou CP, Lewin JM, Chiang CL, et al. Clinical evaluation of contrast-enhanced digital mammography and contrast enhanced tomosynthesis—comparison to contrast-enhanced breast MRI. Eur J Radiol 2015; 84(12):2501–8.

45. Lalji UC, Houben IP, Prevos R, et al. Contrast-enhanced spectral mammography in recalls from the Dutch breast cancer screening program: validation of results in a large multireader, multicase study. Eur Radiol 2016;26(12):4371–9.

46. Saraya S, Adel L, Mahmoud A. Indeterminate breast lesions: can contrast enhanced digital mammography change our decisions? The Egyptian Journal of Radiology and Nuclear Medicine 2017; 48(2):547–52.

47. Tardivel AM, Balleyguier C, Dunant A, et al. Added value of contrast-enhanced spectral mammography in postscreening assessment. Breast J 2016;22(5): 520–8.

48. Houben IP, Vanwetswinkel S, Kalia V, et al. Contrast-enhanced spectral mammography in the evaluation of breast suspicious calcifications: diagnostic accuracy and impact on surgical management. Acta Radiol 2019;60(9):1110–7.

49. Tennant SL, James JJ, Cornford EJ, et al. Contrast-enhanced spectral mammography improves diagnostic accuracy in the symptomatic setting. Clin Radiol 2016;71(11):1148–55.

50. Moustafa AFI, Kamal EF, Hassan MM, et al. The added value of contrast enhanced spectral mammography in identification of multiplicity of suspicious lesions in dense breast. The Egyptian Journal of Radiology and Nuclear Medicine 2018;49(1): 259–64.

51. Cheung YC, Tsai HP, Lo YF, et al. Clinical utility of dual-energy contrast-enhanced spectral mammography for breast microcalcifications without associated mass: a preliminary analysis. Eur Radiol 2016; 26(4):1082–9.

52. Cheung YC, Juan YH, Lin YC, et al. Dual-energy contrast-enhanced spectral mammography: enhancement analysis on BI-RADS 4 non-mass microcalcifications in screened women. PLoS One 2016;11(9):e0162740.

53. Patel BK, Naylor ME, Kosiorek HE, et al. Clinical utility of contrast-enhanced spectral mammography as an adjunct for tomosynthesis-detected architectural distortion. Clin Imaging 2017;46:44–52.

54. Cheung YC, Lin YC, Wan YL, et al. Diagnostic performance of dual-energy contrast-enhanced subtracted mammography in dense breasts compared to mammography alone: interobserver blind-reading analysis. Eur Radiol 2014;24(10): 2394–403.

55. Mori M, Akashi-Tanaka S, Suzuki S, et al. Diagnostic accuracy of contrast-enhanced spectral mammography in comparison to conventional full-field digital mammography in a population of women with dense breasts. Breast Cancer 2017; 24(1):104–10.

56. Zuley ML, Bandos AI, Abrams GS, et al. Contrast Enhanced Digital Mammography (CEDM) helps to safely reduce benign breast biopsies for low to moderately suspicious soft tissue lesions. Acad Radiol 2020;27(7):969–76.

57. Helal MH, Mansour SM, Ahmed HA, et al. The role of contrast-enhanced spectral mammography in the evaluation of the postoperative breast cancer. Clin Radiol 2019;74(10):771–81.

58. Niell BL, Freer PE, Weinfurtner RJ, et al. Screening for breast cancer. Radiol Clin North Am 2017; 55(6):1145–62.

59. Berg WA. Current status of supplemental screening in dense breasts. J Clin Oncol 2016;34(16):1840–3.

60. U.S. Food & Drug Administration. MQSA insights: 2019 scorecard statistics 2020. Available at: https://www.fda.gov/radiation-emitting-products/mqsa-insights/2019-scorecard-statistics. Accessed March 18, 2020.

61. Patel BK, Gray RJ, Pockaj BA. Potential cost savings of contrast-enhanced digital mammography. AJR Am J roentgenology 2017;208(6):W231–7.

62. Jeukens CR, Lalji UC, Meijer E, et al. Radiation exposure of contrast-enhanced spectral mammography compared with full-field digital mammography. Invest Radiol 2014;49(10):659–65.

63. Harvey JA, Anderson RT, Patrie JT, et al. Preferences and attitudes regarding adjunct breast cancer screening among patients with dense breasts. J Breast Imaging 2020;2(2):119–24.

64. Choudhery S, Patel BK, Johnson M, et al. Trends of supplemental screening in women with dense breasts. J Am Coll Radiol 2020;17(8):990–8.

65. Rhodes D, Hunt K, Ellis R, et al. Molecular breast imaging and tomosynthesis to eliminate the reservoir of undetected cancer in dense breasts: the density MATTERS trial. San Antonio (TX): San Antonio Breast Cancer Symposium; 2019.

66. Sung JS, Lebron L, Keating D, et al. Performance of dual-energy contrast-enhanced digital mammography for screening women at increased risk of breast cancer. Radiology 2019;293(1):81–8.

67. Kim G, Phillips J, Cole E, et al. Comparison of contrast-enhanced mammography with conventional digital mammography in breast cancer screening: a pilot study. J Am Coll Radiol 2019; 16(10):1456–63.

68. Sorin V, Yagil Y, Yosepovich A, et al. Contrast-enhanced spectral mammography in women with intermediate breast cancer risk and dense breasts. AJR Am J roentgenology 2018;211(5):W267–74.

69. Melnikow J, Fenton JJ, Whitlock EP, et al. Supplemental screening for breast cancer in women with dense breasts: a systematic review for the U.S. Preventive Services Task Force. Ann Intern Med 2016; 164(4):268–78.

70. Bakker MF, de Lange SV, Pijnappel RM, et al. Supplemental MRI screening for women with extremely dense breast tissue. N Engl J Med 2019;381(22): 2091–102.

71. Comstock CE, Gatsonis C, Newstead GM, et al. Comparison of abbreviated breast MRI vs digital breast tomosynthesis for breast cancer detection among women with dense breasts undergoing screening. JAMA 2020;323(8):746–56.

72. Caro JJ, Trindade E, McGregor M. The risks of death and of severe nonfatal reactions with high- vs low-osmolality contrast media: a meta-analysis. AJR Am J roentgenology 1991;156(4):825–32.

73. Katayama H, Yamaguchi K, Kozuka T, et al. Adverse reactions to ionic and nonionic contrast media. A report from the Japanese Committee on the Safety of Contrast Media. Radiology 1990;175(3):621–8.

74. Luk L, Steinman J, Newhouse JH. Intravenous contrast-induced nephropathy-the rise and fall of a threatening idea. Adv Chronic Kidney Dis 2017; 24(3):169–75.

75. Feig S. Cost-effectiveness of mammography, MRI, and ultrasonography for breast cancer screening. Radiol Clin North Am 2010;48(5):879–91.

76. Covington MF, Young CA, Appleton CM. American College of Radiology accreditation, performance metrics, reimbursement, and economic considerations in breast MR imaging. Magn Reson Imaging Clin N Am 2018;26(2):303–14.

77. Kuhl CK, Schrading S, Strobel K, et al. Abbreviated breast magnetic resonance imaging (MRI): first postcontrast subtracted images and maximum-intensity projection-a novel approach to breast cancer screening with MRI. J Clin Oncol 2014;32(22): 2304–10.

78. Chhor CM, Mercado CL. Abbreviated MRI protocols: wave of the future for breast cancer screening. AJR Am J Roentgenology 2017;208(2):284–9.

79. Burwell SM. Setting value-based payment goals–HHS efforts to improve U.S. health care. N Engl J Med 2015;372(10):897–9.

80. Patel BK, Ranjbar S, Wu T, et al. Computer-aided diagnosis of contrast-enhanced spectral mammography: a feasibility study. Eur J Radiol 2018;98: 207–13.

Is It the Era for Personalized Screening?

Carolina Rossi Saccarelli, MD[a,b], Almir G.V. Bitencourt, MD, PhD[a,c], Elizabeth A. Morris, MD[a,*]

KEYWORDS

- Screening • Breast cancer • High risk • Personalized medicine • Early detection • MR imaging

KEY POINTS

- We live in an era of risk prediction, tailored screening, and personalized treatment.
- It is important to be aware that some current screening recommendations might be driven by cost-effectiveness considerations.
- Individual screening recommendations should be made through a shared decision-making process, enabling women to make an informed decision with their physicians based on their particular risks and priorities.
- Recent advances in breast MR imaging, especially abbreviated protocols, support the increasing use of this method as an excellent alternative to mammography for screening women with higher than average risk.
- Further studies should be performed to ensure the best screening strategy for each specific population.

INTRODUCTION

Breast cancer screening is a recognized tool for early detection of the disease in asymptomatic women, improving treatment efficacy and reducing the mortality rate. Multiple historic randomized controlled trials have demonstrated the benefit of breast cancer screening using mammography.[1–3] A recent Swedish trial, with a population of more than half million women, demonstrated a 41% reduction in the risk of dying from breast cancer in 10 years and a 25% reduction in the rate of advanced breast cancers, in participating women versus those not participating in the screening.[4] Despite the consensus regarding its benefits, the screening recommendations have been widely debated over the past years and controversies remain regarding the optimal screening strategy.[5–7]

Because breast cancers are heterogeneous and have their own particularities,[8,9] each woman is also different with unique risk factors, so the need for breast cancer screening varies from one woman to another.[10,11] Other imaging tools besides mammography, such as digital breast tomosynthesis (DBT), ultrasound (US), and MR imaging, play an important role in supplemental screening, particularly in women with an elevated risk of breast cancer, in whom mammography alone has a lower accuracy.[12,13]

These understandings have raised awareness that a "one-size-fits-all" approach cannot be applied for breast cancer screening. Currently, despite the specific guidelines for a minority of women who are at very high risk of breast cancer (eg, BRCA1, BRCA2, and other known genetic mutation carriers, or patients with strong family history of breast or ovarian cancers), all other women are still treated alike.

This article reviews the current recommendations for breast cancer risk assessment and breast

[a] Breast Imaging Service, Department of Radiology, Memorial Sloan Kettering Cancer Center, 300 East 66th Street, New York, NY 10065, USA; [b] Department of Radiology, Hospital Sírio-Libanês, Rua Dona Adma Jafet 91, São Paulo, SP 01308-050, Brazil; [c] Department of Imaging, A.C. Camargo Cancer Center, Rua Prof. Antônio Prudente, 211, São Paulo, SP 01509-010, Brazil
* Corresponding author.
E-mail address: morrise@mskcc.org

Radiol Clin N Am 59 (2021) 129–138
https://doi.org/10.1016/j.rcl.2020.09.003
0033-8389/21/© 2020 Elsevier Inc. All rights reserved.

radiologic.theclinics.com

cancer screening in average-risk and higher-than-average-risk women, and discusses new developments and future perspectives for personalized breast cancer screening.

BREAST CANCER RISK ASSESSMENT

Breast cancer risk assessment should be performed at a young age because hereditary breast cancer syndromes are associated with early onset breast cancer and patients with these syndromes need tailored screening recommendations. The American College of Radiology (ACR) recommends that breast cancer risk assessment should be performed in all women at the age of 30 years to guide counseling on surveillance, genetic testing, and risk reduction treatments.[14]

In clinical practice, risk assessment is performed with validated statistical tools to calculate the lifetime risk of breast cancer, including Gail, Claus, Tyrer–Cuzick, BRCAPRO, and BOADICEA (Breast and Ovarian Analysis of Disease Incidence and Carrier Estimation) models, which are based on classical risk factors, such as age, family history of breast and ovarian cancer, and personal medical and reproductive history (Table 1). All these models have been validated in specific populations and have limitations; thus, it is important to know which models are not applicable or possibly less accurate for a specific patient.[15] Mathematical risk assessment models also vary in their ability to accurately incorporate risk associated with personal history of high-risk lesions, such as atypical ductal hyperplasia and lobular neoplasia, and most of these models do not include mammographic density assessment, which helps to predict individual risk of breast cancer.[16] Recently, Yala and colleagues[17] showed promising results from deep learning models using mammographic images demonstrating a substantially improved risk assessment compared with an established breast cancer risk model as Tyrer-Cuzick. They also demonstrated increased accuracy with a hybrid deep learning model, which used traditional risk factors and mammogram images, showing an accurate risk assessment model at an individual level, making breast cancer screening more personalized than ever.

Because most available risk assessment models are not applicable to women with hereditary cancer syndromes, it is essential to determine if a patient is a candidate for genetic counseling and genetic testing before being submitted to a breast cancer risk assessment tool. There are also several available tools to guide referral for genetic counseling, including the National Comprehensive Cancer Network (NCCN) guidelines, Ontario Family History Assessment Tool, Manchester Scoring System, and Referral Screening Tool. In general, patients should be considered for genetic counseling if they have a personal or family history of ovarian cancer at any age, breast cancer at 50 years of age or younger, bilateral or triple-negative breast cancer at any age, male breast cancer, or Ashkenazi Jewish heritage. The genetic specialist then determines whether and which genetic testing is appropriate for each patient.[15] Fig. 1 shows a breast cancer risk assessment algorithm.

There is a proliferation of genetic tests being developed for screening; however, genetic testing is still a work in progress. Most genetic testing criteria have been based on the probability of having a pathogenic variant in the BRCA1 and BRCA2 genes, which are high-penetrance genes. However, new technologies have allowed the development of multigene panel tests, which include other individual genes where variants confer a moderate to high risk of breast cancer, such as TP53 (Li-Fraumeni syndrome), PTEN (Cowden syndrome and the Bannayan–Ruvalcaba–Riley–Smith syndrome), CDH1, STK11, BRIP1, PALPB, CHEK2, and ATM.[18]

Although only a small proportion ($\leq$10%) of breast cancers are caused by hereditary mutations in single, dominantly acting genes, currently available evidence suggests that a larger fraction of sporadic breast cancer cases might be attributable to the action of multiple genes.[18] In particular, polygenic risk scores based on low-penetrance single-nucleotide polymorphisms have been shown to play an important role in breast cancer risk assessment and will probably be more broadly used in the future.[19–21] To date, it seems that the polygenic risk score information is actually additive to the information provided by conventional risk assessment tools.[22,23]

SCREENING OF AVERAGE-RISK WOMEN

A woman is considered to be at average-risk if she has 15% or less lifetime risk of breast cancer on risk assessment tools. The American Cancer Society (ACS) considers that an average-risk woman should not have personal history of breast cancer, strong family history of breast cancer, high-risk predisposition syndromes or genetic mutations, or history of thoracic radiation therapy before the age of 30 years.[24] Mammography is still the mainstay of breast cancer screening because it is broadly available, with established quality assurance, and has been tested within prospective randomized trials.[3] In addition, the ACR also states it may be appropriate to consider adding handheld

Table 1
Breast cancer risk assessment models currently used in clinical practice

Model	Personal History of Breast Disease	Personal History of Ovarian Cancer	BRCA Gene	Family History of Breast and Ovarian Cancer	Ashkenazi Inheritance	Breast Density	Hormonal, Reproductive, and Other Factors
BOADICEA v5	Breast cancer	Yes	Yes	First- and second-degree female and male relatives	Yes	Yes	Age of menarche and first live birth, menopause status, HRT, weight
BRCAPRO	Breast cancer	Yes	Yes	First- and second-degree female and male relatives	No	No	Ethnicity
Claus	Breast cancer	Yes	No	First- and second-degree female and male relatives	No	No	No
Gail	ADH, ALH	No	No	First-degree female relatives	No	No	Age of menarche and first live birth, ethnicity
Tyrer-Cuzick v8	ADH, ALH, LCIS	Yes	Yes	First-, second-, and third-degree female relatives; first-degree male relative	Yes	Yes	Age of menarche and first live birth, menopause status, HRT, weight

Abbreviations: ADH, atypical ductal hyperplasia; ALH, atypical lobular hyperplasia; HRT, hormone-replacement therapy; LCIS, lobular carcinoma in situ.

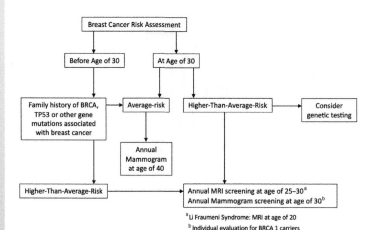

Fig. 1. Algorithm for breast cancer risk assessment.

or automated breast US to mammography in women with dense breasts, thereby increasing the rate of cancer detection weighed against the risk of increasing the false-positive rate significantly with screening US.[2]

Unlike in Europe, where many countries have organized national screening programs,[25,26] the United States has opportunistic screening and many specialty societies publish divergent recommendations regarding the frequency of screening and the age range in which screening should be performed (Table 2).

Although the US Preventive Services Task Force and American College of Physicians recommend biennial mammography for women aged 50 to 74 years,[27,28] the ACR, Society of Breast Imaging, ACS, and NCCN recommend that screening should be performed annually beginning at age 40 years.[1,7] Despite these different recommendations, most societies agree that mammographic screening should be offered at age 40 years for average-risk women and that the benefits and potential harms should be discussed to achieve a personalized screening strategy through a shared decision-making process.

The decision of when to start and how often to perform screening mammography is usually based on each institution's values and on the balance between benefits and perceived harms of screening (ie, overdiagnosis and false-positive results). Annual screening results in fewer deaths from breast cancer, especially in younger women, although it also leads to higher costs associated with additional recalls and invasive procedures.[1,6] Some guidelines (ie, from the American College of Physicians and US Preventive Services Task Force) are based on cost-effectiveness and economic considerations, trying to do a fair allocation of limited health care resources. However, other guidelines are based on the medical and psychological implications of screening. Often missing from these discussions are the reduced costs associated with early detection: identifying cancer at an earlier stage may result in less invasive treatment and decreased morbidity from surgery, chemotherapy, and radiation therapy. In addition, the costs of a late breast cancer diagnosis because of nonscreening, which includes increased treatment-related morbidity and loss of quality-adjusted life-years, may be even higher than the costs of screening. In fact, these nuances should not be decided by societies, but should be decided by women individually with their physician, based on their risk factors and priorities.

There are many reasons to perform breast cancer screening in the 40s. First, breast cancer is an important cause of death in women younger than 50 years of age. The problem, however, is that compared with women older than 50 years of age, women younger than 50 are less likely to develop breast cancer, which increases the number of women needed to screen to avoid one breast cancer death, a common metric used to evaluate screening cost-effectiveness. However, an early diagnosis in women younger than 50 would be even more important because these women tend to develop biologically aggressive rapid-growing cancer, where early diagnosis is of great importance. The social impact of cancer death is higher in the 40s and more than 40% of the years of life lost to breast cancer are in women diagnosed in this age group, not to mention the economic impact to families and societies.[29] Additionally, in some specific racial groups (ie, African-American and Asian women), the peak incidence of breast cancer happens earlier. Thus, the decision based on individual risk of developing breast

Table 2
Recommendations for breast cancer screening in average-risk women

	ACR	NCCN	ACS	ACP, USPSTF	EUSOBI	ESMO
Age to initiate (y)	40	40	45; offer at 40–44	50; individualize at 40–49	50; consider also 40–49	50; consider also 40–49
Screening interval	Annual	Annual	Annual for 40–54; biennial or annual >55	Biennial	Biennial for 50–69; annual for 40–49	Annual or biennial for 50–69
Age to end	Not yet established; continue if life expectancy >5–7 y	Not yet established; continue if life expectancy ≥10 y	Continue if life expectancy ≥10 y	74	69; consider also 70–74	69; consider also 70–74

Abbreviations: ACP, American College of Physicians; ESMO, European Society of Medical Oncology; EUSOBI, European Society of Breast Imaging; USPSTF, US Preventive Services Task Force.

cancer should be more relevant than the decision based on cost-effectiveness.

Breast MR imaging is the most sensitive tool for breast cancer screening, providing a high cancer detection rate (15 per 1000 women). Despite being commonly used for screening in high-risk women, breast MR imaging is not recommended for screening average-risk women, and the main limitations for its widespread use include high cost and limited availability. To reduce the costs associated with image acquisition and image interpretation of screening breast MR imaging, abbreviated protocols have been proposed, which take an acquisition time of less than 10 minutes (compared with 20–30 minutes in the full protocol) with comparable diagnostic accuracy to the full protocol.[30–34]

Recently, two large randomized trials demonstrated the benefits of using breast MR imaging screening in average-risk women with dense breasts. The Dense Tissue and Early Breast Neoplasm Screening (DENSE) trial, a multicenter controlled trial in the Netherlands, randomized more than 40,000 women aged between 50 and 75 years with extremely dense breast tissue and normal results on screening mammography to a group that was invited to undergo supplemental MR imaging or to a group that received mammography screening only. The use of supplemental MR imaging screening in these women resulted in the diagnosis of significantly fewer interval cancers than mammography alone during a 2-year screening period (estimated to be lower by 4.2 per 1000 screenings).[35] The EA1141 trial, a multicenter study conducted by the ECOG-ACRIN Cancer Research Group in the United States and Germany, enrolled 1516 average-risk women aged 40 to 75 years with heterogeneously dense or extremely dense breasts undergoing routine screening. All women underwent screening by DBT and abbreviated breast MR imaging. Abbreviated breast MR imaging was associated with a significantly higher rate of invasive breast cancer detection (11.8 per 1000 women vs 4.8 per 1000 women).[36] Future studies should investigate the results of abbreviated breast MR imaging as a stand-alone breast cancer screening method for all women.

SCREENING OF HIGHER-THAN-AVERAGE-RISK WOMEN

Women with more than 15% lifetime risk of breast cancer on risk assessment tools are considered to be at higher than average risk. These women should undergo different screening strategies, including the use of supplemental imaging

modalities, especially MR imaging.[14,37] MR imaging is the most sensitive imaging test for breast cancer screening and it detects cancers at an earlier stage than mammography.[38] Current evidence supports its use as an effective breast cancer surveillance tool, especially in high-risk populations, given the aggressive behavior and natural history of mutation-associated breast cancers.[39]

The ACS and NCCN guidelines recommend supplemental annual breast MR imaging screening for women at very high risk for breast cancer, which include BRCA mutation carriers and their untested first-degree relatives, women with Li-Fraumeni syndrome and other high-risk predisposition syndromes, women with a history of thoracic radiation therapy (10 Gy or more) between age 10 and 30 years, and women with 20% or greater lifetime risk of breast cancer based on risk-assessment models. Annual MR imaging screening should start at age 25 to 30 and annual mammography screening is also recommended, starting preferably at age 30.[40,41] There is also increasing evidence to support the addition of MR imaging to annual mammography screening in women with a personal history of breast cancer, which improves detection of early stage but biologically aggressive breast cancers with a high specificity.[42–44] The ACR already recommends breast MR imaging annual screening for women with personal history of breast cancer and dense breast tissue, or those diagnosed before age 50.[14] For women with personal history of atypical ductal hyperplasia, atypical lobular hyperplasia, or lobular carcinoma in situ, the ACR suggests that MR imaging should also be considered for screening, especially if other risk factors are present.[14]

The effectiveness of mammography screening in high-risk women has been questioned, especially in young women and in BRCA1/2 carriers, in whom there is particular concern about the risk of radiation-induced breast cancer.[45] This is attributed to the higher breast density and lower sensitivity of mammography in this age group.[46] Prior studies have shown that adding mammography to screening MR imaging did not significantly improve sensitivity in BRCA1/2 carriers younger than age 40 compared with MR imaging alone, suggesting that mammography screening should be reconsidered in this cohort.[47–50]

The EVA trial, a prospective multicenter observational cohort study with 687 high-risk women, demonstrated that mammography plus MR imaging did not add a significant improvement to the cancer yield achieved by quality-assured MR imaging alone performed annually.[51] Besides, MR imaging detects primarily invasive cancers and high-grade ductal carcinoma in situ, whereas most additional cancers detected at screening mammography in this population are lower grade ductal carcinoma in situ.[52,53] However, some authors found that mammography can bring additional value for screening high-risk women older than age 40 years, especially those aged 50 to 69 years, and should be considered as being associated with MR imaging, especially in BRCA2 carriers with dense breasts, who tend to develop breast cancer at an older age compared with BRCA1 carriers.[54] In this population, DBT should be preferred to digital mammography because of the higher rates of screening-detected cancer and lower false-positive recalls.[55]

The best interval period to perform screening MR imaging and the preferred MR imaging protocol are still under debate. It is known that tumors in mutation carriers grow faster than those in average-risk women at the same age.[56] Thus, reducing the screening intervals in the former population may improve screening outcomes for them as long as the screening test used is able to reliably detect these fast-growing tumors. MR imaging's benefit over mammography is that it overcomes the masking effect of dense breasts on mammography. A recent prospective study by Guindalini and colleagues[48] suggested that MR imaging screening every 6 months had a significantly higher specificity rate and similar sensitivity compared with MR imaging plus annual mammography in mutation carriers, especially in BRCA1 carriers. In this intensive surveillance study, the authors also demonstrated that there were no patients with lymph node metastasis at the time of diagnosis and no interval invasive cancers. The disadvantage of biannual MR imaging is the higher cost, which is alleviated with abbreviated MR imaging protocols, which also have high diagnostic accuracy.[34] Breast MR imaging screening using abbreviated breast MR imaging protocol is noninferior to screening with a full protocol and may result in significantly higher screening specificity and shorter reading time.[57]

PERSONALIZED SCREENING AND FUTURE PERSPECTIVES

The American College of Obstetricians and Gynecologists guidelines, published in 2017, stated that average-risk women should be offered screening mammography at age 40 years and that the screening strategy should be made through a shared decision-making process between patient and physician.[58] In this context, women who are willing to undergo screening should be counseled in a way that only addresses the medical issues instead of cost considerations. It is important that the information provided to women about the benefits and potential harms of screening should be available in a transparent and objective way so they can make an informed decision. However, the issues of screening are complex (ie, advantages and disadvantages of different imaging methods) so that it really requires someone with deep knowledge of screening to communicate the benefits and risks. The regular health care provider usually does not have the knowledge and time to discuss these issues. This is a great opportunity for breast radiologists to participate in this shared decision-making process. Furthermore, it may be the radiologists' responsibility to help advocate for the most appropriate imaging for the patient, given their expertise knowledge.

Although significant progress has been made in the last few decades, not only in the biologic heterogeneity of breast cancer, but also in risk prediction tools, not much has been applied in clinical practice to improve breast cancer screening. Different women have different needs for screening because of different risks and beliefs. We are now heading toward a more personalized approach, especially with advances in artificial intelligence, where women considered to be at average risk, according to regular assessment tools, could actually be at greater risk, and they will need an individualized screening strategy with different types and frequency of examinations. Better risk-assessment tools are needed in clinical practice. Additionally, the patient's risk changes over time, and reassessment is needed to be done at regular intervals, rather than just once in a lifetime.

It is hoped that, in the near future, more individualized and accurate risk assessment tools that include classical risk factors, genetic assessment, imaging features, and artificial intelligence could increase patient awareness of lifetime breast cancer risk. Some of these tools, such as assessing mammography texture and density, are close to being used on a wider scale. It is likely that, in the coming years, screening programs will use more personalized tools to improve their outcomes.

SUMMARY

We live in an era of risk prediction, tailored screening, and personalized treatment. It is important to be aware that some of current screening recommendations might be driven by cost-effectiveness considerations. Individual screening recommendations should be made through a shared decision-making process, enabling women to make an informed decision with their physicians based on their particular risks and priorities. Recent advances in breast MR imaging, especially abbreviated protocols, support the increasing use of this method as an excellent alternative to mammography for screening women with higher than average risk. Further studies should be performed to ensure the best screening strategy for each specific population.

CLINICS CARE POINTS

- Breast cancer risk assessment should be performed at a young age because hereditary breast cancer syndromes are associated with early onset breast cancer and patients with these syndromes need tailored screening recommendations.
- Risk models have been validated in specific populations and all have limitations; thus, it is important to know which models are not applicable or possibly less accurate for a specific patient.

DISCLOSURE

E.A. Morris received a grant from Grail, Inc, for research not related to this present article.

REFERENCES

1. Helvie MA, Bevers TB. Screening mammography for average-risk women: the controversy and NCCN's position. J Natl Compr Canc Netw 2018;16(11): 1398–404.
2. Mainiero MB, Moy L, Baron P, et al. ACR Appropriateness Criteria ® Breast Cancer Screening. J Am Coll Radiol 2017;14(11):S383–90.
3. Myers ER, Moorman P, Gierisch JM, et al. Benefits and harms of breast cancer screening. JAMA 2015;314(15):1615.
4. Duffy SW, Tabár L, Yen AM, et al. Mammography screening reduces rates of advanced and fatal breast cancers: results in 549, 091 women. Cancer 2020;1–9. https://doi.org/10.1002/cncr.32859.
5. Witten M, Parker CC. Screening mammography. Surg Clin North Am 2018;98(4):667–75.
6. Eby PR. Evidence to support screening women annually. Radiol Clin North Am 2017;55(3):441–56.
7. Lee CS, Moy L, Friedewald SM, et al. Harmonizing breast cancer screening recommendations: metrics and accountability. Am J Roentgenol 2018;210(2): 241–5.
8. Rivenbark AG, O'Connor SM, Coleman WB. Molecular and cellular heterogeneity in breast cancer. Am J Pathol 2013;183(4):1113–24.
9. Ellsworth RE, Blackburn HL, Shriver CD, et al. Molecular heterogeneity in breast cancer: state of the science and implications for patient care. Semin Cell Dev Biol 2017;64:65–72.
10. Carney PA, Miglioretti DL, Yankaskas BC, et al. Individual and combined effects of age, breast density, and hormone replacement therapy use on the accuracy of screening mammography. Ann Intern Med 2003;138(3):168–75.
11. Tilanus-Linthorst M, Verhoog L, Obdeijn I-M, et al. A BRCA1/2 mutation, high breast density and prominent pushing margins of a tumor independently contribute to a frequent false-negative mammography. Int J Cancer 2002;102(1):91–5.
12. Houssami N, Lord SJ, Ciatto S. Breast cancer screening: emerging role of new imaging techniques as adjuncts to mammography. Med J Aust 2009;190(9):493–7. Available at: http://www.ncbi. nlm.nih.gov/pubmed/19413520.
13. Takahashi TA, Lee CI, Johnson KM. Breast cancer screening: does tomosynthesis augment mammography? Cleve Clin J Med 2017;84(7):522–7.
14. Monticciolo DL, Newell MS, Moy L, et al. Breast cancer screening in women at higher-than-average risk: recommendations from the ACR. J Am Coll Radiol 2018;15(3):408–14.
15. Barke LD, Freivogel ME. Breast cancer risk assessment models and high-risk screening. Radiol Clin North Am 2017;55(3):457–74.
16. Lee CI, Chen LE, Elmore JG. Risk-based breast cancer screening: implications of breast density. Med Clin North Am 2017;101(4):725–41.
17. Yala A, Lehman C, Schuster T, et al. A deep learning mammography-based model for improved breast cancer risk prediction. Radiology 2019;292(1):60–6.
18. Foulkes WD. Inherited susceptibility to common cancers. N Engl J Med 2008;359(20):2143.
19. Wood ME, Farina NH, Ahern TP, et al. Towards a more precise and individualized assessment of breast cancer risk. Aging (Albany NY) 2019;11(4): 1305–16.
20. Piccinin C, Panchal S, Watkins N, et al. An update on genetic risk assessment and prevention: the role of genetic testing panels in breast cancer. Expert Rev Anticancer Ther 2019;19(9):787–801.
21. Mavaddat N, Pharoah PDP, Michailidou K, et al. Prediction of breast cancer risk based on profiling with common genetic variants. J Natl Cancer Inst 2015; 107(5). https://doi.org/10.1093/jnci/djv036.
22. Cuzick J, Brentnall AR, Segal C, et al. Impact of a panel of 88 single nucleotide polymorphisms on the risk of breast cancer in high-risk women: results from two randomized tamoxifen prevention trials. J Clin Oncol 2017;35(7):743–50.
23. Zhang X, Rice M, Tworoger SS, et al. Addition of a polygenic risk score, mammographic density, and endogenous hormones to existing breast cancer

risk prediction models: a nested case–control study. PLoS Med 2018;15(9):e1002644. Zheng W, editor.

24. Oeffinger KC, Fontham ETH, Etzioni R, et al. Breast cancer screening for women at average risk: 2015 Guideline update from the American Cancer Society. JAMA 2015;314(15):1599–614.

25. Sardanelli F, Aase HS, Álvarez M, et al. Position paper on screening for breast cancer by the European Society of Breast Imaging (EUSOBI) and 30 national breast radiology bodies from Austria, Belgium, Bosnia and Herzegovina, Bulgaria, Croatia, Czech Republic, Denmark, Estonia, Finland, France, G. Eur Radiol 2017;27(7):2737–43.

26. Cardoso F, Kyriakides S, Ohno S, et al. Early breast cancer: ESMO Clinical Practice Guidelines for diagnosis, treatment and follow-up. Ann Oncol 2019. https://doi.org/10.1093/annonc/mdz173.

27. Siu AL. Screening for breast cancer: U.S. Preventive Services Task Force Recommendation Statement. Ann Intern Med 2016;164(4):279.

28. Qaseem A, Lin JS, Mustafa RA, et al. Screening for breast cancer in average-risk women: a guidance statement from the American College of Physicians. Ann Intern Med 2019;170(8):547.

29. Ray KM, Price ER, Joe BN. Evidence to support screening women in their 40s. Radiol Clin North Am 2017;55(3):429–39.

30. Kuhl CK. Abbreviated breast MRI for screening women with dense breast: the EA1141 trial. Br J Radiol 2018; 91(1090). https://doi.org/10.1259/bjr.20170441.

31. Ko ES, Morris EA. Abbreviated magnetic resonance imaging for breast cancer screening: concept, early results, and considerations. Korean J Radiol 2019; 20(4):533–41.

32. Kuhl CK. Abbreviated magnetic resonance imaging (MRI) for breast cancer screening: rationale, concept, and transfer to clinical practice. Annu Rev Med 2019;70(1):501–19.

33. Partovi S, Sin D, Lu Z, et al. Fast MRI breast cancer screening: ready for prime time. Clin Imaging 2020; 60(2):160–8.

34. Leithner D, Moy L, Morris EA, et al. Abbreviated MRI of the breast: does it provide value? J Magn Reson Imaging 2018;1–16. https://doi.org/10.1002/jmri. 26291.

35. Bakker MF, De Lange SV, Pijnappel RM, et al. Supplemental MRI screening for women with extremely dense breast tissue. N Engl J Med 2019;381(22): 2091–102.

36. Comstock CE, Gatsonis C, Newstead GM, et al. Comparison of abbreviated breast MRI vs digital breast tomosynthesis for breast cancer detection among women with dense breasts undergoing screening. JAMA 2020;323(8):746–56.

37. Mann RM, Kuhl CK, Moy L. Contrast-enhanced MRI for breast cancer screening. J Magn Reson Imaging 2019. https://doi.org/10.1002/jmri.26654.

38. Saadatmand S, Geuzinge HA, Rutgers EJT, et al. MRI versus mammography for breast cancer screening in women with familial risk (FaMRIsc): a multicentre, randomised, controlled trial. Lancet Oncol 2019;20(8):1136–47.

39. Obdeijn IM, Winter-Warnars GAO, Mann RM, et al. Should we screen BRCA1 mutation carriers only with MRI? A multicenter study. Breast Cancer Res Treat 2014;144(3):577–82.

40. Saslow D, Boetes C, Burke W, et al. American Cancer Society guidelines for breast screening with MRI as an adjunct to mammography. Obstet Gynecol Surv 2007;62(7):458–60.

41. Clinical N, Guidelines P, Guidelines N. Genetic/familial high-risk assessment: breast and ovarian. J Natl Compr Canc Netw 2018;8(5):562–94.

42. Cho N, Han W, Han B-K, et al. Breast cancer screening with mammography plus ultrasonography or magnetic resonance imaging in women 50 years or younger at diagnosis and treated with breast conservation therapy. JAMA Oncol 2017;3(11): 1495–502.

43. An YY, Kim SH, Kang BJ, et al. Feasibility of abbreviated magnetic resonance imaging (AB-MRI) screening in women with a personal history (PH) of breast cancer. PLoS One 2020;15(3):e0230347.

44. Houssami N, Cho N. Screening women with a personal history of breast cancer: overview of the evidence on breast imaging surveillance. Ultrasonography 2018;37(4):277–87.

45. Pijpe A, Andrieu N, Easton DF, et al. Exposure to diagnostic radiation and risk of breast cancer among carriers of BRCA1/2 mutations: retrospective cohort study (GENE-RAD-RISK). BMJ 2012; 345(7878):1–15.

46. Riedl CC, Luft N, Bernhart C, et al. Triple-modality screening trial for familial breast cancer underlines the importance of magnetic resonance imaging and questions the role of mammography and ultrasound regardless of patient mutation status, age, and breast density. J Clin Oncol 2015;33(10): 1128–35.

47. Phi XA, Houssami N, Hooning MJ, et al. Accuracy of screening women at familial risk of breast cancer without a known gene mutation: individual patient data meta-analysis. Eur J Cancer 2017;85: 31–8.

48. Guindalini RSC, Zheng Y, Abe H, et al. Intensive surveillance with biannual dynamic contrast-enhanced magnetic resonance imaging downstages breast cancer in BRCA1 mutation carriers. Clin Cancer Res 2019;25(6):1786–94.

49. van Zelst JCM, Mus RDM, Woldringh G, et al. Surveillance of women with the BRCA 1 or BRCA 2 mutation by using biannual automated breast US, MR imaging, and mammography. Radiology 2017; 285(2):376–88.

50. Krammer J, Pinker-Domenig K, Robson ME, et al. Breast cancer detection and tumor characteristics in BRCA1 and BRCA2 mutation carriers. Breast Cancer Res Treat 2017;163(3):565–71.

51. Kuhl C, Weigel S, Schrading S, et al. Prospective multicenter cohort study to refine management recommendations for women at elevated familial risk of breast cancer: the EVA Trial. J Clin Oncol 2010; 28(9):1450–7.

52. Sung JS, Stamler S, Brooks J, et al. Breast cancers detected at screening MR imaging and mammography in patients at high risk: method of detection reflects tumor histopathologic results. Radiology 2016; 280(3):716–22.

53. Kuhl CK, Schrading S, Bieling HB, et al. MRI for diagnosis of pure ductal carcinoma in situ: a prospective observational study. Lancet 2007; 370(9586):485–92.

54. Phi XA, Greuter MJW, Obdeijn IM, et al. Should women with a BRCA1/2 mutation aged 60 and older be offered intensified breast cancer screening? A cost-effectiveness analysis. Breast 2019;45:82–8.

55. Hofvind S, Hovda T, Holen ÅS, et al. Digital breast tomosynthesis and synthetic 2D mammography versus digital mammography: evaluation in a population-based screening program. Radiology 2018;287(3):787–94.

56. Tilanus-Linthorst MMA, Obdeijn IM, Hop WCJ, et al. BRCA1 mutation and young age predict fast breast cancer growth in the Dutch, United Kingdom, and Canadian magnetic resonance imaging screening trials. Clin Cancer Res 2007;13(24):7357–62.

57. van Zelst JCM, Vreemann S, Witt H-J, et al. Multireader Study on the diagnostic accuracy of ultrafast breast magnetic resonance imaging for breast cancer screening. Invest Radiol 2018;53(10):579–86.

58. Committee on Practice Bulletins—Gynecology. Practice Bulletin Number 179: Breast Cancer Risk Assessment and Screening in Average-Risk Women. Obstet Gynecol 2017;130(1):e1-e16.

Applications of Artificial Intelligence in Breast Imaging

Matthew B. Morgan, MD, MS[a],*, Jonathan L. Mates, MD[b,1]

KEYWORDS

- Breast imaging • Artificial intelligence • Machine learning • Mammography

KEY POINTS

- The use of AI in radiology has great potential to improve patient safety and clinical outcomes.
- Breast imaging is an attractive target for AI given the relevant clinical problem, the algorithmic nature of the workflow, the narrow focus of the disease process, and the reliance on imaging data.
- Although image analysis and interpretation will be useful, noninterpretive tasks will also benefit from AI technology.
- Leveraging the strengths of both human and machine will likely produce the best value, but only if the AI tools are adequately validated with prospective studies and designed with human interaction and workflow in mind.

INTRODUCTION

Artificial intelligence (AI) is a cross-disciplinary field in which computer scientists, mathematicians, and engineers work to create algorithms that "learn" to take complex inputs and deliver outputs faster and more accurately than the human mind. Although some AI scientists imagine creating the most humanlike machine possible (general AI), most recent work has focused on areas in which AI can perform a specific task (narrow AI).

The recent availability of large digital datasets (big data) combined with improved hardware (graphical processing units or GPUs) has made AI applications into a practical reality. One of the key approaches powered by these advances is machine learning (ML). Whereas early AI consisted of distilling human thought and behavior into discrete steps that can be programmed as clear instructions, ML uses statistical models to allow computer systems to learn and improve without explicit programming.

In the past few years, AI has propelled into the public consciousness and common usage, spreading dramatically into all facets of our lives, including security surveillance (facial recognition), personal assistants (Siri, Alexa), self-driving cars (Google, Uber), financial bots (high-frequency trading, fraud detection), and countless others.

An intense interest in the use of AI in image recognition began in approximately 2009 when a massive dataset was created (ImageNet) and researchers competed in various challenges to evaluate algorithms designed for large-scale object detection and image classification.[1] These successes led to an explosion in the interest of using these techniques to facilitate medical image diagnosis.

ML systems may use imaging features not evident to human perception. This raises the exciting possibility that AI could someday not only make imaging more efficient, but achieve quality improvements such as more reliable diagnoses than what is possible by humans alone.

[a] Department of Radiology and Imaging Sciences, University of Utah, 50 North Medical Drive, Salt Lake City, UT 84132, USA; [b] Viz.ai, San Francisco, CA, USA
[1] Present address: 3000 Danville Boulevard Suite F #312, Alamo, CA 94507.
* Corresponding author.
E-mail address: mbmrad@gmail.com

Radiol Clin N Am 59 (2021) 139–148
https://doi.org/10.1016/j.rcl.2020.08.007
0033-8389/21/© 2020 Elsevier Inc. All rights reserved.

Breast imaging, with its focus on a single diagnosis determined almost exclusively by imaging, represents an ideal use-case for AI efforts in radiology. Screening mammography is particularly well-suited to development of AI applications given the standardized views, comparison images, and robust outcome data, all of which support the training of AI systems.

Breast Cancer Screening

The strengths and limitations of screening mammography will be familiar to breast imagers. Screening mammography is one of the most successful tools for early breast cancer detection and has been shown to decrease mortality.[2–4] Despite its relative success, screening mammography is still far from perfect, with up to 13% of cancers missed at time of interpretation.[4] Approximately 10% of women who undergo breast screening each year are recalled for additional diagnostic imaging, whereas only a small fraction (~5%) of these women are eventually diagnosed with breast cancer.[4] The high rate of false positive screening recalls may lead to patient anxiety and unnecessary biopsies, and add to annual mammography screening costs.[5] If AI technology could help to reduce false positives and simultaneously increase cancer detection rates, it would be a significant improvement to the breast cancer screening process.

Computer-Aided Detection

Computer-aided detection (CAD) is a generic term that refers to the approach of using computers to assist the radiologist to identify a potentially significant finding on an image. The idea of using computers to aid in the mammographic detection process is not new. From the late 1980s through the late 1990s, significant efforts were made to use quantitative analysis of mammography images to identify suspicious lesions such as clustered microcalcifications, masses, and architectural distortions.[6,7]

In 1998, The Food and Drug Administration (FDA) approved the first CAD technology (Image-Checker; Hologic, Bedford, MA) for mammography.[8] When the Centers for Medicare and Medicaid Services (CMS) provided increased payment for its use in 2002, CAD was widely adopted by the breast imaging community, and by 2012 its use in screening exceeded 80%.[9]

However, despite the early promise of improved performance, subsequent research showed that the use of this type of CAD was associated with decreased accuracy and increased biopsy rate.[9,10] Although it continues to be a feature in many mammography systems, early CAD is viewed by many as a failure.[11,12] The reason is that early CAD algorithms suffer from a high false positive rate. To put this in perspective, the average number of CAD marks per full examination ranges from 1.5 to 5.1.[13–15] Assuming 2 marks per examination and added detection of 0.1 to 1 cancer per 1000 examinations, this translates to 1 in 2000 to 20,000 marks as true positives. With this high rate of "false alarms," it is likely that radiologists have learned to largely ignore the CAD markings.

This early version of CAD used human-driven, rule-based mathematical models to determine the presence of abnormal imaging features and could not subsequently improve with additional inputs. Recent advances in ML have opened up a new line of techniques for CAD that offer advantages over prior approaches, thereby creating an opportunity to revisit the idea of CAD for mammography as well as other breast imaging modalities.[16]

In this article, we first briefly review the breast imaging workflow to illustrate the many decision points and show where AI technologies may be applied. We then move to a discussion of the value proposition of AI in breast imaging, its evaluation and limitations, and plausible near-term applications. The intent is to point industry toward the most fruitful use-cases and to provide a framework for breast imagers who are looking to adopt AI into their practice.

BREAST IMAGING WORKFLOW

Breast imaging workflow consists of multiple steps, which can be subdivided into 4 stages: pre-screening, screening, diagnostic, and management (Fig. 1). At each stage, there are decision points that guide the next steps in the workflow. A careful understanding of these decision points can serve as a roadmap for how AI technology could be applied to the breast imaging process.

APPLICATIONS OF ARTIFICIAL INTELLIGENCE

We have summarized the opportunities for AI enhancement of breast imaging in Table 1.

Interpretive Artificial Intelligence

Screening triage
Radiologists review screening mammograms looking for signs of cancer, including masses, architectural distortions, and microcalcifications. This process is essentially a triage to decide if the patient requires further investigation and has 2 basic outcomes: "normal" (Breast Imaging-

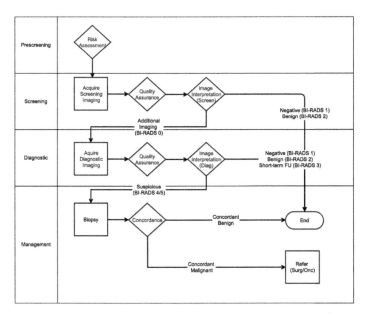

Fig. 1. A process diagram to illustrate the breast imaging workflow. There are 4 stages including prescreening, screening, diagnostics, and management. AI technology may be applied at various process steps (*squares*) and decision points (*diamonds*) to enhance the clinical decision-making process. For organizational purposes, these are grouped into 2 categories: (1) interpretive (*red*), and (2) noninterpretive (*blue*).

Reporting and Data System [BI-RADS] 1 & 2) and "possibly abnormal" (BI-RADS 0). Although this seems straightforward, there is high variability in reader performance[17] with high rates of false positive recalls and a significant number of false negatives (ie, missed cancers).[4] AI technology could improve the screening process in several ways.

Although there is much excitement in proving that a computer could reliably detect cancer, another more pragmatic function could be to reliably identify the negative and benign cases.[18–20] Recent research has shown that differentiating "normal" exams (BI-RADS 1 & 2) from the "possibly abnormal" exams (BI-RADS 0) could reduce the overall number of cases that require human review by 15% to 20%.[20] These normal results could be shared immediately, which would

decrease overall anxiety for patients awaiting test results.[20,21]

Screening AI could decrease reader variance by helping radiologists with different levels of training and experience achieve more uniform performance.

AI systems could also serve as stand-alone second readers in screening programs in which double reads are performed.[20,22]

Although much attention is focused on 2-dimensional screening mammography, other screening modalities such as tomosynthesis, ultrasound, and MR imaging would also benefit from AI development. Because these use more images per study than mammography, the use of AI could potentially result in efficiency gains with equal or improved quality.[23]

Artificial intelligence–based computer-aided detection

After triage, AI could be leveraged in screening to help detect areas of concern (AI-based CAD). This is where the bulk of current AI research is focused, and numerous recent studies have shown promising results.[24–33] The combination of human review with AI-based CAD would be synergistic for making final determinations on examination recalls, which should simultaneously decrease recall rates while improving cancer detection rates.

At the diagnostic imaging stage, the imaging task shifts from lesion detection to lesion characterization and risk stratification for potential biopsy. Additional mammographic views and/or ultrasound are used to isolate the abnormality

Table 1
Applications for artificial intelligence (AI) in breast imaging include interpretive and noninterpretive tasks

Interpretive AI	Noninterpretive AI
Screening triage	Risk assessment
AI-based computer-aided detection	Imaging controls
	Scan acquisition and reconstruction
	Dose reduction
	Quality assurance
	Radiologic-pathologic correlation
	Workflow optimization

and allow for detailed feature analysis. AI in this setting would become a tool to analyze the region of interest identified by radiologists to characterize its features. This would increase overall accuracy (positive predictive value [PPV] of biopsy) and decrease intraobserver and interobserver variation by decreasing the impact of differences in training and experience. AI could also be used as a "second reader" to help validate radiologists' impressions.[34,35]

More advanced uses might include detecting features not visible to humans and advanced statistical analysis. Research is under way to predict cancer based on enhancement features,[36] predict cancer subtypes and genomics,[37] predict response to treatment,[38–41] and assess lymph nodes for signs of spread.[42–45]

Noninterpretive Artificial Intelligence

Although much of the focus of AI in mammography has been on image analysis and interpretation, there are many noninterpretive aspects of the breast cancer workflow that would benefit from AI.[46,47]

Risk assessment

Before any imaging takes place, the first step in the cancer screening process should be to understand a woman's individual cancer risk. Accurate risk analysis can then help guide the initiation of screening, frequency, and optimal modality(ies).

Without risk analysis, mammography screening guidelines necessarily lump all women together. This overgeneralization has produced differing recommendations of when to begin screening and at what frequency,[48–50] with the resultant controversy creating a confusing message for women and their primary care providers.[51]

To help improve screening personalization, several breast cancer risk models have incorporated patient-specific characteristics such as age, family history, and hormonal factors to refine breast cancer risk estimation.[52–55] Mammographic breast density was recently added to risk models, and legislation in many US states requires that women be notified of their breast density with the well-meaning intent of informing them about the decreased sensitivity of mammography in dense breasts and helping them understand the impact on breast cancer risk. However, density assessment suffers from significant interreader variability, which may cause confusion if the density is assessed differently year to year.[55,56] Moreover, the focus on density may result in overemphasis of a single factor in risk, rather than improving overall risk estimation.

A recent study has shown that AI analysis of mammography (without including traditional risk factors) can significantly improve breast cancer risk prediction, which would be especially helpful when family history is unknown.[57,58] The same research shows that when AI image analysis is *combined* with traditional risk model information, performance increases further still. Such improvements would allow each woman to have a personalized and data-driven approach to breast screening, with screening commencement and frequency adjusted accordingly. This approach could help to mitigate the controversy from overgeneralized, age-based screening recommendations.

Image controls

Applying AI in the image acquisition process has the potential to improve patient safety, image quality, process efficiency, and technologist performance.

Dose reduction

The ALARA principle ("As Low As Reasonably Achievable") is familiar to radiologists. Radiation dose is especially relevant to a screening examination that is repeated over many years. One of the major potential benefits of AI in breast imaging would be to reduce the dose without compromising image quality. Novel techniques are being tested that could maintain high image quality while dose is reduced by up to 50%.[59,60]

Quality assurance

Because the features of cancer on imaging may be subtle, high-quality imaging is critical. In the United States, rigorous imaging standards are required by the Mammography Quality Standards Act and the American College of Radiology.[61,62] Image evaluation includes an assessment of positioning, compression, artifacts, exposure, contrast, sharpness, noise, and labeling.

In the current mammography workflow, a radiologist makes a subjective assessment of image quality at the time of interpretation. If it does not meet quality standards, a "technical recall" is issued and the patient must return for inconvenient and wasteful repeat imaging. From a Lean manufacturing principles standpoint, quality problems should be detected and corrected at the time of acquisition or prevented altogether.

ML algorithms that automatically assess the image quality could be built into the image acquisition process. This way, blur and/or positioning problems can be detected while the patient is still in the room and can be re-imaged with minimal increased effort.

AI applied to mammography quality assurance would reduce or even eliminate technical recalls and improve technologist performance by giving just-in-time feedback. It could also facilitate accreditation by automatically identifying high-quality images. Moreover, AI could assess overall system performance by retrospective image review to identify potential quality improvement initiatives.

Radiologic-pathologic correlation (and beyond)

After a biopsy, breast imagers review the pathologic result and compare it with the imaging appearance to determine "radiology-pathology correlation." This is a manual process and is subject to significant variability in decisions and management, especially when results include "high-risk" pathologies. AI could standardize the decision making by incorporating quantitative imaging features, semantic features of the radiology and pathology reports, histopathologic slide imaging features, as well as patient risk factors.

Moreover, there is growing evidence that *imaging* has potential use in understanding *genomic* properties of disease.[60] Radiomics is an approach that extracts features from radiographic images using data-characterization algorithms, which may uncover disease characteristics humans are unable to perceive. Radiogenomics refers to the relationship between the digital pattern in disease imaging (imaging phenotype), and its genetic expression, including gene mutations and other genome-related characteristics.[63] The combination of radiogenomics with AI tools could provide a powerful approach for uncovering radiologic-pathologic-genomic relationships and increasing prognostic potential.[64]

Workflow optimization

In emergency radiology, AI is being used to help prioritize studies with urgent positive findings, such as intracranial hemorrhage, pulmonary embolism, spinal fracture, and others.[65,66] This new approach to organizing and prioritizing examinations could be leveraged in breast imaging as well. AI-identified normal examinations could be overread in an expedited fashion (or given an AI-only reading) to give immediate results. Examinations flagged with probable abnormalities could be prioritized for immediate diagnostic evaluation, or they could be concentrated for review at the beginning of the day when radiologist attention is fresh and before image fatigue.[67] Examinations with very high probability cancers could automatically trigger workflows that could alert care coordinators and preschedule a diagnostic examination, biopsy appointment, and prompt surgical consultation.

DISCUSSION

Integrating Artificial Intelligence

Humans and machines have different strengths; the goal of AI in health care should be to leverage the advantages of both.

Some tasks are better suited for computers. Machines never get tired. They produce consistent and repeatable results. They can "see" what humans cannot, analyzing data beyond the limits of human perception and at remarkable speed. Machines excel at pattern recognition, even those involving large volumes of data with complex associations, and can therefore provide improved predictive power.

Humans, on the other hand, can synthesize disparate points of data. We can make inferences from minimal data and solve a wide variety of problems. Humans can incorporate context, adapt to regional practice patterns or other idiosyncratic situations, build working relationships, and clearly communicate with referring clinicians and patients. Humans can extract value and meaning from the vast store of unstructured and messy information that is the current state of medical data.

In breast imaging, there are numerous points of correlation, judgment, procedural skill, assessment, and communication with both patient and referring clinician. Clearly, AI is not a replacement for these high-level, highly nuanced tasks. Although the introduction of AI has often been cast as a struggle between humans and machines, the true power of AI will be realized when it is incorporated in a way that harmonizes the skill of humans with the power of technology using an interface that optimizes that synthesis and allows for iterative feedback. Lack of this harmonization and feedback is likely one of the reasons why traditional CAD failed to meet expectations.[68]

As we consider how to integrate AI into practice, it may be instructive to compare with other industries. For example, the automotive industry has identified 6 levels of automation to describe the process of integrating AI into the driving process. In breast imaging, we might use a similar paradigm to understand when and how to bring AI into the process (**Fig. 2**).

Although it may be interesting and instructive to imagine the different levels of automation in breast imaging, it is important to keep in mind that the progression to ever-increasing automation is not a foregone conclusion. Automation may remain at a lower level due to reasons of quality plateaus, diminishing returns of value, or even lack of business incentives.

It is also important to note that the progression to higher levels of automation will require

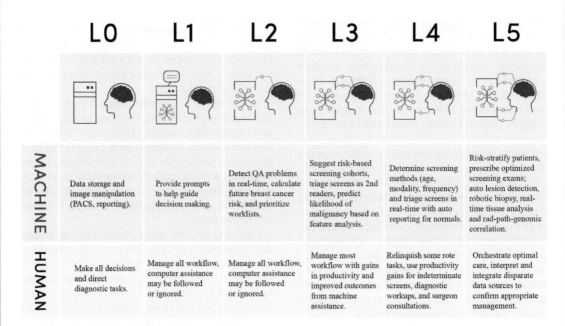

Fig. 2. The 6 levels of AI automation. Level 0 (L0) = no automation, L1 = simple assistance, L2 = partial automation, L3 = conditional automation, L4 = high automation, and L5 = highest automation. PACS, Picture Archiving and Communications System; QA, quality assurance.

increasing degrees of trust. Just as buying a car without a steering wheel would cause apprehension, automating medical decision making should create a similar unease. The humans in the process (patients, physicians, payors, regulatory officials) will need to trust the systems and the organizations developing them. This will require trustworthy processes in the development of AI applications, such as rigorous training and validation, extensive publication of results, and honest business practices. Trust is also a product of repeated positive experiences over time, thus the more AI applications provide transparency in their results, add clear value, and are easy to use, the more trust will be engendered.

VALUE PROPOSITION

The goal of any new technology is to provide value. Despite controversy over implementing screening guidelines, the current breast imaging process has evolved into a thoughtful methodology based on evidence and careful consideration. If AI is to be introduced into the process, it will need to prove its value along the standard value axes.

Increased Efficiency

Radiologists are constantly striving to do more in less time. Even after years of streamlining the breast imaging workflow, there is still potential to relieve radiologists of repetitive tasks in which their cognitive skills add less value. AI can auto-categorize tissue density, locate areas of interest, and pre-populate reports to give radiologists a "head start" on the reporting process. After proper clinical trials and strong evidence is in place, AI could reduce screening workload by auto-reporting normal examinations. Offloading these types of tasks to a computer could allow radiologists to spend more time on more cognitive work, facilitating their ability to practice at the "top of their license."

Improved Quality

To know if AI improves quality and consistency, the AI proof will be in the audit pudding. Audit reports will need to show decreased recall rates, increased PPVs, decreased tumor sizes, and increased cancer detection rates. The fact that the breast imaging process already tracks this "scorecard" data makes proving the benefit of AI relatively straightforward.

Cost Savings/Revenue Generation

It is realistic to consider that within a few years, AI could be shown to consistently identify normal screening examinations with a confidence that matches or exceeds current human performance. If some percentage of screening examinations can be accurately auto-classified and reported as normal without direct human interpretation, then this would translate to a cost reduction for screening interpretation. Further savings may be realized if AI assistance reduces false negatives, and therefore, malpractice payouts.

Beyond cost savings, revenue generation is an important effect in the United States, where health care operates in a largely fee-for-service paradigm. If financial incentives are introduced to encourage use of AI, such as when CMS approved an additional charge for use of CAD, then we can expect widespread adoption of AI technology.

EVALUATION

Implementation of AI in clinical practice will require clearing of several major hurdles, including making sure it works (performance validation), helping the user understand how it works (trust), and integrating it into workflow (user experience design).

Performance Validation

AI algorithm performance can be assessed using standard statistical measures, the detailed discussion of which is beyond the scope of this article. Yet, like the scientific literature in general, it behooves radiologists to be conversant with these concepts and how to read the data.[69]

Preliminary research has necessarily used retrospective data sets in constrained settings to show the potential capabilities of AI in detection and classification. However, before AI can be fully embraced for patient care, it must be tested in prospective trials with patients who fulfill predefined eligibility criteria for the target population to prove there are no issues with bias or transferability. In addition, multi-institutional, well-curated data sets sponsored by national organizations would be helpful to facilitate creation of more robust models for testing and validation in the clinical setting.

Trust

Trusting tools to make crucial decisions will be difficult without the ability to show the rationale followed. This is what is known as the "black box" problem of AI. This is problematic not only for lack of transparency, but also for possible biases inherited by the algorithms. Human prejudices and possible artifacts hidden in the training data may lead to unfair or wrong decisions.[70] This black box problem is a well-known issue in the AI world, and radiologists should require that vendors seek to mitigate it as much as possible.

Conversely, it will be just as important to guard against too much reliance on AI. Evidence shows that human nature is quick to take cognitive shortcuts.[71] We must avoid "dependence lock-in" in which people's deepening dependence on machine-driven networks will erode their ability to think for themselves.[72] AI tools should be used only so long as we can trust humans to overrule them when necessary.

User Experience Design

Even an accurate and trusted AI system will fail if it does not perform well within the context of the clinical workflow and the human-computer interaction.[73] Research methodology tends to remove human factors for the sake of simplicity and convenience. Yet, to be successful, these systems must be designed so that humans and machines solve tasks jointly, and their evaluation should depend on the success of the machine as a tool in the larger process.[74]

SUMMARY

We believe that breast imaging has the potential to be at the vanguard of AI use in medical imaging given the relevant clinical problem, the algorithmic nature of the workflow, the narrow focus of the disease process, and the reliance on imaging data. AI technology can add value in both image interpretation and noninterpretive tasks, and has great potential to improve patient safety and clinical outcomes. Success will require that AI tools are not only validated with prospective studies but also designed to fit into the workflow and leverage the strengths of both humans and machines.

ACKNOWLEDGMENTS

The author acknowledges Michael Mozdy for his assistance in figure and table preparation.

DISCLOSURE

M.B. Morgan, consultant at Elsevier, Inc. No relevant conflicts of interest and no funding sources for this article. J.L. Mates, employee at Viz.ai. No relevant conflicts of interest and no funding sources for this article.

REFERENCES

1. Deng J, Dong W, Socher R, et al. ImageNet: a large-scale hierarchical image database. 2009 IEEE Conference on Computer Vision and Pattern Recognition. Miami (FL), June 20-25, 2009. DOI: 10.1109/CVPR.2009.5206848.
2. Elmore JG, Armstrong K, Lehman CD, et al. Screening for breast cancer. JAMA 2005;293(10): 1245–56.

3. Nelson HD, Cantor A, Humphrey L, et al. Screening for breast cancer: a systematic review to update the 2009 U.S. Preventive Services Task Force recommendation. Rockville (MD): Agency for Healthcare Research and Quality (US); 2016.

4. Lehman CD, Arao RF, Sprague BL, et al. National performance benchmarks for modern screening digital mammography: update from the breast cancer surveillance consortium. Radiology 2017; 283(1):49–58.

5. O'Donoghue C, Eklund M, Ozanne EM, et al. Aggregate cost of mammography screening in the United States: comparison of current practice and advocated guidelines. Ann Intern Med 2014;160(3):145.

6. Chan HP, Doi K, Galhotra S, et al. Image feature analysis and computer-aided diagnosis in digital radiography. I. Automated detection of microcalcifications in mammography. Med Phys 1987;14(4): 538–48.

7. Doi K, Giger ML, Nishikawa RM, et al. Computer-aided diagnosis of breast cancer on mammograms. Breast Cancer 1997;4(4):228–33.

8. U.S. Food and Drug Administration. Premarket Approval (PMA). 1998. Available at: https://www.accessdata.fda.gov/scrIpts/cdrh/cfdocs/cfpma/pma.cfm?id=P970058. Accessed March 3, 2020.

9. Lehman CD, Wellman RD, Buist DSM, et al. Diagnostic accuracy of digital screening mammography with and without computer-aided detection. JAMA Intern Med 2015;175(11):1828–37.

10. Fenton JJ, Taplin SH, Carney PA, et al. Influence of computer-aided detection on performance of screening mammography. N Engl J Med 2007; 356(14):1399–409.

11. Kohli A, Jha S. Why CAD failed in mammography. J Am Coll Radiol 2018;15(3 Pt B):535–7.

12. Bahl M. Detecting breast cancers with mammography: will AI succeed where traditional CAD failed? Radiology 2019;290(2):315–6.

13. Cole EB, Zhang Z, Marques HS, et al. Impact of computer-aided detection systems on radiologist accuracy with digital mammography. AJR Am J Roentgenol 2014;203(4):909–16.

14. Baker JA, Rosen EL, Lo JY, et al. Computer-aided detection (CAD) in screening mammography: sensitivity of commercial CAD systems for detecting architectural distortion. AJR Am J Roentgenol 2003;181(4):1083–8.

15. Scaranelo AM, Eiada R, Bukhanov K, et al. Evaluation of breast amorphous calcifications by a computer-aided detection system in full-field digital mammography. Br J Radiol 2012;85(1013):517–22.

16. Kohli M, Prevedello LM, Filice RW, et al. Implementing machine learning in radiology practice and research. AJR Am J Roentgenol 2017;208(4): 754–60.

17. Barlow WE, Chi C, Carney PA, et al. Accuracy of screening mammography interpretation by characteristics of radiologists. J Natl Cancer Inst 2004; 96(24):1840–50.

18. Aboutalib SS, Mohamed AA, Berg WA, et al. Deep learning to distinguish recalled but benign mammography images in breast cancer screening. Clin Cancer Res 2018;24(23):5902–9.

19. Yala A, Schuster T, Miles R, et al. A deep learning model to triage screening mammograms: a simulation study. Radiology 2019;293(1):38–46.

20. Rodriguez-Ruiz A, Lång K, Gubern-Merida A, et al. Can we reduce the workload of mammographic screening by automatic identification of normal exams with artificial intelligence? A feasibility study. Eur Radiol 2019;29(9):4825–32.

21. Johnson AJ, Easterling D, Nelson R, et al. Access to radiologic reports via a patient portal: clinical simulations to investigate patient preferences. J Am Coll Radiol 2012;9(4):256–63.

22. Mahase E. AI system outperforms radiologists in first reading of breast cancer screening, study claims. BMJ 2020;368:m16.

23. Conant EF, Toledano AY, Periaswamy S, et al. Improving accuracy and efficiency with concurrent use of artificial intelligence for digital breast tomosynthesis. Radiol Artif Intell 2019;1(4):e180096.

24. Rodríguez-Ruiz A, Krupinski E, Mordang J-J, et al. Detection of breast cancer with mammography: effect of an artificial intelligence support system. Radiology 2019;290(2):305–14.

25. Le EPV, Wang Y, Huang Y, et al. Artificial intelligence in breast imaging. Clin Radiol 2019;74(5):357–66.

26. Houssami N, Kirkpatrick-Jones G, Noguchi N, et al. Artificial intelligence (AI) for the early detection of breast cancer: a scoping review to assess AI's potential in breast screening practice. Expert Rev Med Devices 2019;16(5):351–62.

27. Mayo RC, Kent D, Sen LC, et al. Reduction of false-positive markings on mammograms: a retrospective comparison study using an artificial intelligence-based CAD. J Digit Imaging 2019;32(4):618–24.

28. Rodriguez-Ruiz A, Lång K, Gubern-Merida A, et al. Stand-alone artificial intelligence for breast cancer detection in mammography: comparison with 101 radiologists. J Natl Cancer Inst 2019;111(9): 916–22.

29. Geras KJ, Mann RM, Moy L. Artificial intelligence for mammography and digital breast tomosynthesis: current concepts and future perspectives. Radiology 2019;293(2):246–59.

30. McKinney SM, Sieniek M, Godbole V, et al. International evaluation of an AI system for breast cancer screening. Nature 2020;577(7788):89–94.

31. Pisano ED. AI shows promise for breast cancer screening. Nature 2020;577(7788):35–6.

32. Kim H-E, Kim HH, Han B-K, et al. Changes in cancer detection and false-positive recall in mammography using artificial intelligence: a retrospective, multi-reader study. Lancet Digit Health 2020. https://doi.org/10.1016/S2589-7500(20)30003-0.

33. Schaffter T, Buist DSM, Lee CI, et al. Evaluation of combined artificial intelligence and radiologist assessment to interpret screening mammograms. JAMA Netw Open 2020;3(3):e200265.

34. van Zelst JC, Tan T, Mann RM, et al. Validation of radiologists' findings by computer-aided detection (CAD) software in breast cancer detection with automated 3D breast ultrasound: a concept study in implementation of artificial intelligence software. Acta Radiol 2020;61(3):312–20.

35. McKinney SM, Sieniek M, Godbole V, et al. International evaluation of an AI system for breast cancer screening. Nature 2020;577(7788):89–94. https://doi.org/10.1038/s41586-019-1799-6.

36. Ji Y, Li H, Edwards AV, et al. Independent validation of machine learning in diagnosing breast cancer on magnetic resonance imaging within a single institution. Cancer Imaging 2019;19(1):64.

37. Ha R, Mutasa S, Karcich J, et al. Predicting breast cancer molecular subtype with MRI dataset utilizing convolutional neural network algorithm. J Digit Imaging 2019;32(2):276–82.

38. Lo Gullo R, Eskreis-Winkler S, Morris EA, et al. Machine learning with multiparametric magnetic resonance imaging of the breast for early prediction of response to neoadjuvant chemotherapy. Breast 2020;49:115–22.

39. Mani S, Chen Y, Li X, et al. Machine learning for predicting the response of breast cancer to neoadjuvant chemotherapy. J Am Med Inform Assoc 2013;20(4):688–95.

40. Mani S, Chen Y, Arlinghaus LR, et al. Early prediction of the response of breast tumors to neoadjuvant chemotherapy using quantitative MRI and machine learning. AMIA Annu Symp Proc 2011;2011:868–77.

41. Tahmassebi A, Wengert GJ, Helbich TH, et al. Impact of machine learning with multiparametric magnetic resonance imaging of the breast for early prediction of response to neoadjuvant chemotherapy and survival outcomes in breast cancer patients. Invest Radiol 2019;54(2):110–7.

42. Dietzel M, Baltzer PAT, Dietzel A, et al. Application of artificial neural networks for the prediction of lymph node metastases to the ipsilateral axilla - initial experience in 194 patients using magnetic resonance mammography. Acta Radiol 2010;51(8):851–8.

43. Zhang Q, Suo J, Chang W, et al. Dual-modal computer-assisted evaluation of axillary lymph node metastasis in breast cancer patients on both real-time elastography and B-mode ultrasound. Eur J Radiol 2017;95:66–74.

44. Zhou L-Q, Wu X-L, Huang S-Y, et al. Lymph node metastasis prediction from primary breast cancer US images using deep learning. Radiology 2020;294(1):19–28.

45. Liu J, Sun D, Chen L, et al. Radiomics analysis of dynamic contrast-enhanced magnetic resonance imaging for the prediction of sentinel lymph node metastasis in breast cancer. Front Oncol 2019;9:980.

46. Richardson ML, Garwood ER, Lee Y, et al. Noninterpretive uses of artificial intelligence in radiology. Acad Radio 2020. https://doi.org/10.1016/j.acra.2020.01.012.

47. Lakhani P, Prater AB, Hutson RK, et al. Machine learning in radiology: applications beyond image interpretation. J Am Coll Radiol 2018;15(2):350–9.

48. Siu AL, U.S. Preventive Services Task Force. Screening for breast cancer: U.S. preventive services task force recommendation statement. Ann Intern Med 2016;164(4):279–96.

49. Monticciolo DL, Newell MS, Hendrick RE, et al. Breast cancer screening for average-risk women: recommendations from the ACR commission on breast imaging. J Am Coll Radiol 2017;14(9):1137–43.

50. Oeffinger KC, Fontham ETH, Etzioni R, et al. Breast cancer screening for women at average risk: 2015 guideline update from the American Cancer Society. JAMA 2015;314(15):1599–614.

51. Haas JS, Sprague BL, Klabunde CN, et al. Provider attitudes and screening practices following changes in breast and cervical cancer screening guidelines. J Gen Intern Med 2016;31(1):52–9.

52. Gail MH, Brinton LA, Byar DP, et al. Projecting individualized probabilities of developing breast cancer for white females who are being examined annually. J Natl Cancer Inst 1989;81(24):1879–86.

53. Claus EB, Risch N, Thompson WD. The calculation of breast cancer risk for women with a first degree family history of ovarian cancer. Breast Cancer Res Treat 1993;28(2):115–20.

54. Tyrer J, Duffy SW, Cuzick J. A breast cancer prediction model incorporating familial and personal risk factors. Stat Med 2004;23(7):1111–30.

55. Brentnall AR, Harkness EF, Astley SM, et al. Mammographic density adds accuracy to both the Tyrer-Cuzick and Gail breast cancer risk models in a prospective UK screening cohort. Breast Cancer Res 2015;17(1):147.

56. Sprague BL, Conant EF, Onega T, et al. Variation in mammographic breast density assessments among radiologists in clinical practice: a multicenter observational study. Ann Intern Med 2016;165(7):457–64.

57. Dembrower K, Liu Y, Azizpour H, et al. Comparison of a deep learning risk score and standard mammographic density score for breast cancer risk prediction. Radiology 2019;294(2):265–72.

58. Sitek A, Wolfe JM. Assessing cancer risk from mammograms: deep learning is superior to conventional risk models. Radiology 2019;292(1):67–8.

59. Cong W, Shan H, Zhang X, et al. Deep-learning-based breast CT for radiation dose reduction. In: Müller B, Wang G, editors. Developments in x-ray tomography XII. San Diego (CA): SPIE; 2019. p. 54. https://doi.org/10.1117/12.2530234.

60. Qadir SA, Zarshenas A, Yang L, et al. Radiation dose reduction in digital breast tomosynthesis (DBT) by means of neural network convolution (NNC) deep learning. In: Krupinski EA, editor. 14th international workshop on breast imaging (IWBI 2018). Atlanta (GA): SPIE; 2018. p. 15. https://doi.org/10.1117/12.2317789.

61. Mammography Quality Standards Act and Program | FDA. Available at: https://www.fda.gov/radiation-emitting-products/mammography-quality-standards-act-and-program. Accessed May 12, 2020.

62. Complete Accreditation Information: Mammography (Revised 12-12-19): Accreditation Support. Available at: https://accreditationsupport.acr.org/support/solutions/articles/11000063274-complete-accreditation-information-mammography. Accessed May 12, 2020.

63. Mazurowski MA. Radiogenomics: what it is and why it is important. J Am Coll Radiol 2015;12(8):862–6.

64. Ashraf AB, Daye D, Gavenonis S, et al. Identification of intrinsic imaging phenotypes for breast cancer tumors: preliminary associations with gene expression profiles. Radiology 2014;272(2):374–84.

65. Arbabshirani MR, Fornwalt BK, Mongelluzzo GJ, et al. Advanced machine learning in action: identification of intracranial hemorrhage on computed tomography scans of the head with clinical workflow integration. NPJ Digit Med 2018;1:9.

66. Annarumma M, Withey SJ, Bakewell RJ, et al. Automated triaging of adult chest radiographs with deep artificial neural networks. Radiology 2019;291(1):196–202.

67. Krupinski EA, Berbaum KS, Caldwell RT, et al. Long radiology workdays reduce detection and accommodation accuracy. J Am Coll Radiol 2010;7(9):698–704.

68. Nishikawa RM, Bae KT. Importance of better human-computer interaction in the era of deep learning: mammography computer-aided diagnosis as a use case. J Am Coll Radiol 2018;15(1 Pt A):49–52.

69. Park SH, Han K. Methodologic guide for evaluating clinical performance and effect of artificial intelligence technology for medical diagnosis and prediction. Radiology 2018;286(3):800–9.

70. Guidotti R, Monreale A, Ruggieri S, et al. A survey of methods for explaining black box models. ACM Comput Surv 2018;51(5):1–42.

71. Tversky A, Kahneman D. Judgment under uncertainty: heuristics and biases. Science 1974;185(4157):1124–31.

72. Anderson J, Rainie L, Luchsinger A. Artificial intelligence and the future of humans. Pew Research Center; 2018. Available at: https://www.pewresearch.org/internet/2018/12/10/artificial-intelligence-and-the-future-of-humans/. Accessed May 13, 2020.

73. Beede E, Baylor E, Hersch F, et al. A human-centered evaluation of a deep learning system deployed in clinics for the detection of diabetic retinopathy. In: Proceedings of the 2020 CHI Conference on Human Factors in Computing Systems. New York: ACM; 2020:1-12. https://doi.org/10.1145/3313831.3376718.

74. Shah NH, Milstein A, Bagley PhD SC. Making machine learning models clinically useful. JAMA 2019. https://doi.org/10.1001/jama.2019.10306.

Moving?

Make sure your subscription moves with you!

To notify us of your new address, find your **Clinics Account Number** (located on your mailing label above your name), and contact customer service at:

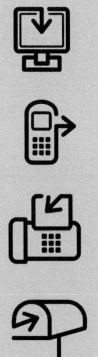

Email: **journalscustomerservice-usa@elsevier.com**

800-654-2452 (subscribers in the U.S. & Canada)
314-447-8871 (subscribers outside of the U.S. & Canada)

Fax number: 314-447-8029

Elsevier Health Sciences Division
Subscription Customer Service
3251 Riverport Lane
Maryland Heights, MO 63043

ELSEVIER

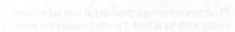

Printed and bound by CPI Group (UK) Ltd, Croydon, CR0 4YY

08/05/2025

01864694-0013